CRISPR EXPLAINED
- Joy and Horror

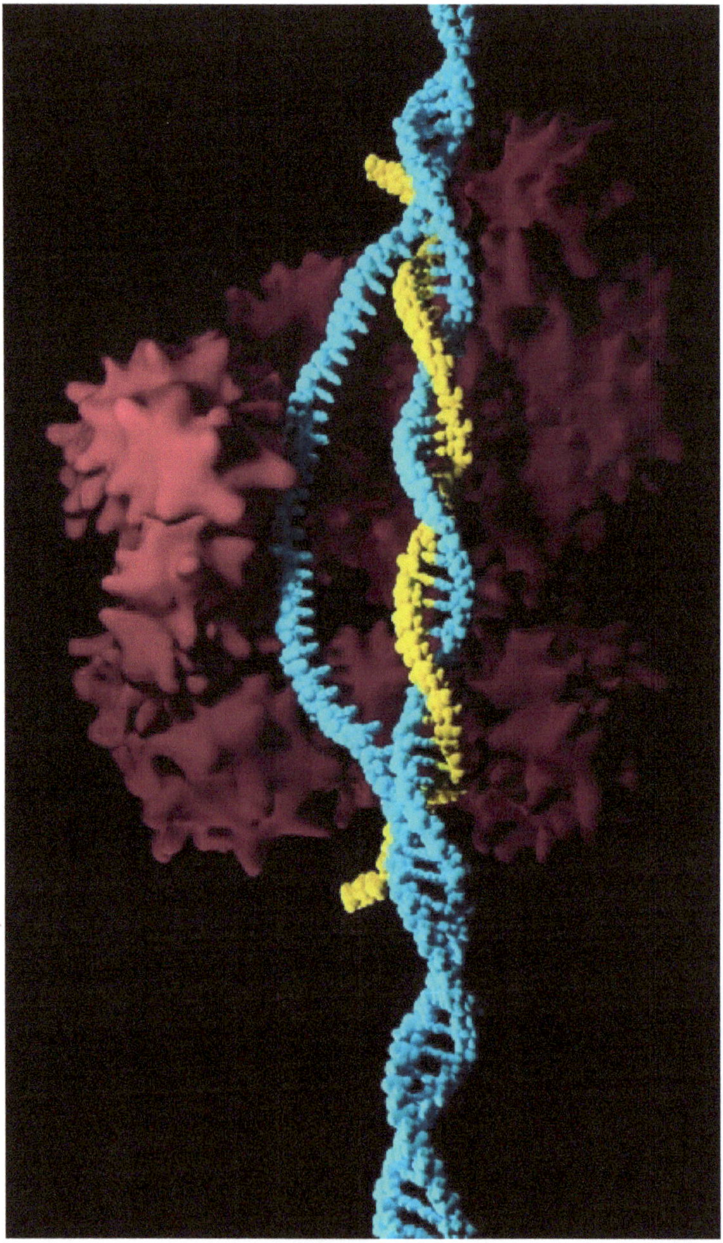

by Fred Dungan

Published and Formatted by DUNGAN BOOKS

ISBN 978-1-63684-181-6
No animals were hurt in the production of this novel.
For my granddaughter, Caitlin

Prologue

Redder, riper tomatoes with a longer shelflife, corn with an extra gene added for sweetness, seedless tangerines, plumper seedless grapes that will stay fresh for months on end, disease resistant vegetables that have been grown without pesticides, future generations of humans born free of sickle cell anemia, rheumatoid arthritis and all other inherited (genetic) diseases—these are but a few of the improvements made possible by Twenty-First Century CRISPR (gene editing).

CRISPR is a tool. In itself CRISPR is neither good nor evil. The purpose that people put it to determines its ethical nature. [For example: a shovel can be used to plant potatoes or misused to knock someone over the head from behind.]

Rumors have been circulating on social media that Covid-19 is a manmade virus created in a laboratory located in Wuhan, China. Whether the rumor is fact or fiction is not within the scope of this book. What is important is that it is possible for someone with an elementary knowledge of Biology to create a virus that could result in a pandemic (or worse). That scares the bejesus out of me.

Introduction

CRISPR is an acronym which stands for clustered regularly interspaced short palindromic repeats. CRISPR technology is a simple yet powerful tool for editing genomes. It allows researchers to easily alter DNA sequences and modify gene function. Its many potential applications include correcting genetic defects, treating and preventing the spread of diseases, and improving crops. However, its promise also raises ethical concerns about whether science should be making permanent changes in the creative process.

One moral concern is that editing DNA creates gene drives. These are genetic systems which increase the chances of a particular trait passing on from parent to offspring. Eventually, over the course of generations, the trait spreads through entire populations. Alter enough DNA in an effort to improve human beings and geneticists could bring about the extinction of our species, much as Cro-Magnon man replaced Neanderthal man, but over a much shorter period of time. I predict that in the not-so-distant future our species, *Homo Sapiens* will be replaced by an improved species which for the sake of clarity, I am labeling *Homo Aurelius*. This will not necessarily be a tragedy since we all desire our descendants to live a better life than we had. As we travel into space and spread our seed throughout the Universe, we will continue to improve our genetic makeup, becoming immortal omnipotent beings ("gods," if you will).

Perhaps civilization's greatest concern about CRISPR is that it is difficult to regulate. Any above average high school Biology student could learn its technique. Gene editing kits are being offered on the internet for as little as $150. In the wrong hands CRISPR could potentially be misused to create apocalyptic designer diseases as destructive (or more destructive) than the plagues that an angry God visited on Biblical Egypt.

In popular usage, "CRISPR" is shorthand for "CRISPR-Cas9." CRISPRs are specialized stretches of DNA. The protein Cas9 (or "CRISPR-associated") is an enzyme that acts like a pair of molecular scissors, capable of cutting strands of DNA.

CRISPR technology was adapted from the natural defense mechanisms of bacteria and archaea (the domain of single-celled microorganisms). These organisms use CRISPR-derived RNA and various Cas proteins, including Cas9, to foil attacks by viruses and other foreign bodies. They do so primarily by chopping up and destroying the DNA of a foreign invader. When these components are transferred into other, more complex, organisms, it allows for the manipulation of genes, or "editing."

The following manuscript was written to dramatically present both the good and the bad sides of the controversy over CRISPR. Does CRISPR need to be regulated? That decision is yours to make. Because I was born an optimist, it is my opinion that the good that CRISPR can do for mankind will ultimately outweigh the bad.

Fred Dungan

Arlington District, Riverside, CA

December 11, 2019

PART I

CRISPR JOY

CHAPTER 1

The Whyte Clinic was founded by Dr. Thomas J. Whyte and eight other prominent geneticists whose black and white portraits hung in gilded frames on the west wall of the Board Room on the top floor of the Whyte Clinic. In 2006 they had collectively felt the need for a facility dedicated to research on DNA and the treatment of inherited diseases. By pooling their resources, together with a generous grant from the Centers for Disease Control, they were able to construct, staff, equip, and open the facility in less than a year, a remarkable achievement for a group of men and women who had known one another primarily by reputation prior to endorsing Dr. Whyte's proposal.

Five of the founders had since then passed away, their places on the Board of Directors taken by four younger geneticists and a Nobel Prize winning epidemiologist. To be seated at the long mahogany table in the Board Room where the Board of Directors held its meetings on the second Thursday of the month was an honor in itself.

CEO and Chairman of the Board, eighty-nine year old Dr. Thomas J. Whyte, gaveled the meeting to order. Dr. Whyte began by asking if there was any old business that needed to be discussed. Encountering silence from the Board, Dr. Whyte announced that the Chairman recognized Dr. Sills, the Chief Financial Officer, who would now give the Board his monthly report.

"Good morning ladies and gentlemen of the Board. This has been a relatively profitable month (and I might add an excellent quarter, financially speaking) for the Whyte Clinic. Income continues to exceed expenditures. There is nothing in the foreseeable future to indicate a downturn such as we had in 2008 – 2009. Hospital bed occupancy fluctuates daily with a monthly mean of 70 percent, a figure comparable to the healthcare industry average. Are there any suggestions as to how we might increase earnings? Dr. Whyte and I have agreed that we need the Board's input on this matter."

Dr. Elizabeth Rand, the epidemiologist, raised her left hand, and having been given the floor, commented "I am new to the Board, so I am not familiar with what has gone on previously, however, I cannot help but wonder why the Whyte Clinic does not advertise its services. Being unique in our field, I envision a nationwide campaign that would put the Whyte Clinic on par with healthcare institutions such as the Mayo Clinic and City of Hope. Let's shoot for a 100 percent occupancy rate."

"Is it ethical and legal for professional institutions to advertise their services and, if so, are there any restrictions on how we go about it?," Dr. Sills asked in an effort to determine the efficacy of Dr. Rand's suggestion.

"Of course it is," Dr. Whyte intervened, "Doctors and

lawyers advertise regularly. The only difference between them and other businesses is that professionals are held to a higher standard. Unlike some questionable enterprises, they cannot get away with making false claims or selling quack cures."

"Yes," Dr. Rand reiterated, "we need to tastefully market our services. Let the public know that we specialize in the eradication of inherited diseases. A woman and her spouse's DNA can be edited to give birth to healthier, more intelligent babies. We can assist clients in choosing the qualities they want their children to have. We can truthfully, and in all good conscience, say that the Whyte Clinic is improving humankind one child at a time. What parent does not want his or her child to succeed? We, fellow members of the Board, are in an enviable position in that we are marketing a service that people would give almost anything to have. Our job is to make them aware of it. I propose using the $2.3 million surplus we carried over from last year to fund an advertising budget for the remainder of this fiscal year."

"I second the motion," declared Dr. Whyte. "All in favor say 'aye.' Those opposing the measure say 'no.' The 'ayes' have it, the measure has passed unanimously." (short pause) "If there are no objections, I hereby appoint Dr. Sill and Dr. Rand to a committee that will decide how best our advertising budget can be spent. The committee will write a report and submit it to me before our next Board meeting."

CHAPTER 2

"You wanna diamond necklace, I go and buy you a diamond necklace," stated Dominic Tavaglione. "You wanna wedding, I go and buy you a frilly white dress—lacey like a fancy French restaurant's tablecloth—and a wannabe Elvis marries us in a glitzy Las Vegas chapel. You want it, I go and buy it, but you ain't getting a kid—that's human trafficking, that will get me 20 to life. I don't deal in drugs or human beings. You wanna kid, you get him the same way anybody else does; dim the lights, put on a Frank Sinatra album, we pop the cork on a magnum of pink champagne, and follow the urge to merge. It's not like it's hard to do. You afraid of ugly stretch marks? Nowadays, doctors do wonders. I heard they can even guarantee a baby's sex and hair color. And it's legit."

"Since when did my Mr. Slick give a hoot about the law? You have yet to earn your first honest dollar," said Mrs. Tavaglione. "Adopting a child has nothing to do with human trafficking. "No one is going to arrest you for rescuing a child from the horrors of the foster care system."

"Go, do what you want to do. Go see a social worker, make an appointment with a doctor. No matter what I say, you always end up getting your way," Dominic complained. "Why should today be different than any other day? The past becomes the present just as the present passes on into the future. Why ask me for my opinion, if you have already decided what you are going to do?"

***

After completing the health history and financial responsibility questionnaire a medical assistant had given her, she took a seat in the waiting room of the Whyte Clinic. Most of the staff and a few of the patients wore disposable face masks to keep from catching an Asian flu virus which had already infected a substantial percentage of the population. Mrs. Tavaglione was not the least bit concerned. She had confronted and prevailed against muggers, buggers, and thieves. She had inherited the .25 caliber nickle-plated pistol in her purse from her late aunt's estate. The women in her family were notoriously aggressive. She had no fear of falling victim to a, God forbid!, ***foreign*** virus.

***

Dr. Owen Ostrowski was seven months out of medical school. He had opted to do his residency at the Whyte Clinic because it stood at the leading edge of DNA/stem cell technology on the West Coast. Hardly a month ever passed by without at least one of its many research teams having published either an article, an update, or a review in a major medical journal.

However, prestige didn't do diddlysquat to pay Dr. Ostrowski's bills. His $50,000 first year residency salary sounded good, but not having much experience with money management, it simply drove him deeper in debt. Saddled with over $475,000 in student loans, what had initially looked like a bright future in medicine was now looking rather bleak. A paralegal informed him that student loans were seldom forgiven nor would they automatically be erased by declaring bankruptcy. Today, Owen was receiving Overdue Bill reminders from his bank. Tomorrow, he feared, it would metastasize into harassing phone calls from collection agencies. He desperately needed a salary hike. There would be an $8,000 increase in his second year of residency. Good, but not nearly enough for Dr. Ostrowski to extricate himself from an insurmountable mountain of debt.

The Country Club lifestyle portrayed on television that doctors purportedly live, had provided the motivation for Owen to become a physician. Now, it was all crumbling before him. Dr. Ostrowski could not qualify to buy a new car, much less a new house. Financially speaking, he would have been better off if he had gone to work in an automobile assembly plant instead of going to medical college.

However, Owen Ostrowski was not entirely without blame for his financial predicament. The loans had been so easy to get that it was tempting to use them for other purposes. When a group of third year medical students spent their summer vacation in Maui, he decided to go with them. The price tag for his frolic was $6,500. Graduation was celebrated by riding his motorcycle through Chernobyl. Why Chernobyl? At the time, it seemed like a daring thing to do. The Russian border guards who arrested him thought otherwise. He was deported to the United States after paying a $2,500 fine.

***

"Carmella Tavaglione," called a nurse from an open doorway. Mrs. Tavaglione stood up stiffly and walked towards the nurse who pointed to a long, narrow hallway and said "third door on the left." After weighing Carmella, the nurse took her pulse, blood pressure , and height, then left the exam room, stating, "Dr. Ostrowski will be with you shortly."

Fifteen minutes later, there came a knock on the exam room door and in stepped a tall, slender physician in a white lab coat.

"Good morning, Mrs. Tavaglione. I am Dr. Ostrowski. It says in your file that this is your first visit to the Whyte Clinic. What can we do for you today?"

"I saw an advertisement from the Whyte Clinic which claimed parents could choose the sex, eye color, and other features that their babies will be born with. I would like to know more about it," Carmella requested.

"We have a tool called CRISPR that can edit DNA, removing unwanted genes and replacing them with wanted genes which are then spliced onto the chromosome much like editors do with film - editing out the bad scenes and replacing them with good scenes. I should warn you that most insurance policies do not cover this procedure," Dr. Ostrowski affirmed. "Each additional change adds both to the price and the chance that something might go wrong."

"At what point does my husband enter into this," queried Mrs. Tavaglione.

"As soon as possible. It would speed up matters if you brought him with you to your next appointment," Dr. Ostrowski replied. "Also, everyone needs to be on the same page. Hopefully, you can reach a consensus. You can influence your family's future—for the next generation and infinite generations to come. DNA never forgets."

"My husband is of the opinion that pre-determining an infant's characteristics was part of the failed Eugenics experimentation that led to Nazi doctors being executed as war criminals at the Nuremberg trials," Carmella postured. "To him, that isn't a bad thing—my husband, Dominic has delusions of founding a new dynasty. Personally, I have no desire to ruin a gorgeous body that cost hundreds of hours and thousands of dollars to create by turning it into a baby factory."

Dr. Ostrowski opened a drawer of his desk and took out some brochures which he handed to Mrs. Tavaglione, commenting "these will help your family to reach a consensus about which qualities you would like for your baby to have, keeping in mind that the editing procedure is rather expensive and involves a small degree of risk. Are there any other issues that we need to discuss?"

"Yes," answered Carmella Tavaglione, "it all seems wrong to me. God determines a baby's sex, hair color, height, blood type, and everything else about him. Now, a lab technician is going to contravene God's orders. That is blasphemy!"

"I wouldn't say that. God brings order to chaos. DNA is little more than a random assembly of proteins. By bringing useful order to DNA, lab technicians are doing good deeds designed to enhance the natural order of things. God does not want you to sit on your behind and whine. Get up and do something to make life better. Future generations will celebrate what we are doing," Dr. Ostrowski rebutted. "Some might argue that using CRISPR technology to edit DNA is tantamount to playing God. Nothing could be further from the truth. Scientists are humans. They are fallible, but they learn from their mistakes and move on."

"I will bring my husband to our next appointment," promised Carmella. "He's rather Old School."

***

In the two week period between Carmella's initial appointment and the follow-up appointment in which Dominic would be included, Mr. and Mrs. Tavaglione studied the Whyte Clinic's brochures and used them to determine the characteristics they most desired in a child. At first they couldn't reach agreement, but with time their disagreement became less emotional. They wrote a detailed description of the ideal child they had in mind. Dominic commented that "it's a bit like deciding which options to take on a new car, only it's a helluva lot more expensive."

***

"Here, Doc," uttered Dominic Tavaglione as he handed Doctor Ostrowski a sheet of yellow lined paper, headlined in Block Letters: 'OUR PERFECT CHILD.' "This is what me and the Missus agreed upon."

"You want a blue-eyed, blonde boy," stated Dr. Ostrowski as he covered the points written in painstakingly perfect longhand cursive almost as if it had been printed in a scripted font. "You also want him to be more than six feet tall at maturity, strongly built, wavy haired, above average intelligence, olive skinned, aquiline nosed, night-visioned, thick wrists, disease immune, Catholic with a humungous, fourteen inch penis. I do not think we can make him religious, but I am rather certain we can edit his DNA in such a way as to produce the rest. My question to you is do you really want to go to the enormous expense of having the perfect child or are you willing to accept something slightly less?"

"Money is no object when it comes to creating a deserving heir," Mrs. Tavaglione countered. "My husband is fully capable of acquiring vast sums of currency. I would rather spend it on this than to squander it on gambling and cheap thrills."

"We just threw in the part about the penis as a last minute item," Dominic interrupted. "We thought it would make life somewhat easier for him."

"No problem," answered Dr. Ostrowski, "did you want fourteen inches at birth or at maturity? Flaccid or aroused?"

"All I meant about the fourteen inches is that I want my kid to be well hung. No wimps or *palomitas* in the Tavaglione Family. Not that there is anything wrong with alternate persuasions, it's just that Fruit Loops and Tavagliones don't mix. Besides, I am the one footing the bill, so what I say matters, kapish?"

"An associate of mine read a letter in Playboy Forum that said the more we alter DNA in our offspring, the more we run the risk of bringing about our own extinction," Dominic claimed. "It said that we, Homo Sapiens, would eventually not be able to breed with those of us with improved DNA, Homo Aurelius, at which point we would go the way of the dodo."

Dr. Ostrowski shook his head before replying, "There is

one minor consolation. A small percentage of our DNA comes from extinct Neanderthals, in fact, some of our DNA can be traced back to each and every step of the evolutionary process, even to when we were one cell organisms billions of years ago. It's called Legacy DNA. Our descendants will always carry a small part of us with them. Rather than vanish, we will simply fade, fade away. But that is conjecture about the distant future, what you need to do is to take care of present business. I'm going to turn you over to a nurse who will take a sperm sample from Mr. Tavaglione. She will also have you sign an authorization form. Afterwards, the Medical Assistant at the front desk will handle the financial arrangements and scheduling your next appointment with me. Also, Mrs. Tavaglione will have to make an appointment for harvesting several eggs. I know that the DNA editing procedure can seem overly long. Your safety and that of the unborn child are of utmost importance here at the Whyte Clinic. Do you have any more questions? If not, I will see Carmella Tavaglione again in three weeks." Dr. Ostrowski shook hands with the soon-to-be-expectant couple and left the exam room shortly after introducing them to his nurse, Ms. Nit.

***

Nurse Nit conducted the Tavagliones to a nearby restroom, gave Dominic a small plastic bottle, and directed him to bring back a sperm sample.

"I'm sor-r-ry, I can-n't," stammered Dominic nervously, "No damn wankers in my family."

"What the . . .?" exclaimed Carmella. Then, addressing Nurse Nit, she asked, "Does this restroom lock from the inside?"

"I believe so," the nurse responded.

"I'll go in with him," Carmella stated authoritatively. "Wait here. This won't take long. I'll be back in five shakes with a sample."

True to her word, Carmella entered the restroom, locked the door, and ordered Dominic to drop his pants. Carmella proved herself a professional. Quickly taking charge, she obtained a sticky sample sometime between the fourth and fifth shake of her deft left palm.

***

Five weeks later, surgeons implanted a DNA edited embryo into Carmella's womb. Eight weeks following the implant, an ultrasound detected three heartbeats, indicating that Carmella would give birth to triplets.

"This happens sometimes in cases where the expectant mother took fertility drugs to get pregnant," the ultrasound technician explained.

It was a difficult pregnancy, but Carmella was able to carry all three fetuses full term. She gave birth to three identical boys, each with blonde hair, blue eyes, and above average height. Of particular interest was an outsized penis, a characteristic which all three shared in common.

CHAPTER 3

Lynda Alvarez's vision slowly deteriorated following her birth to the point where a physician declared her legally blind seven months after her sixth birthday. She had been diagnosed with Leber congenital amaurosis, a disease which grew steadily worse until now on the eve of her 23rd birthday her world was one big blur—her sole comfort was that she could still tell light from dark.

Lynda's mother was busy in the kitchen, baking a chocolate cake and preparing guacamole for tomorrow's birthday party which for the most part would be attended by relatives and a few close friends.

Actually, the party was more for Lynda's mother than it was for Lynda. One of the consequences of being disabled is that the afflicted person, having, through no fault of their own, become dependent on others, frequently continues to be treated like a child long after attaining the age of majority even when their impairment is physical rather than mental. Lynda knew from past experience that it would be a child's birthday party—no alcohol, tobacco, or—heaven forbid—sex permitted. All that would be missing would be the hired clown and that was only because that role was reserved for Lynda (or so she felt). She longed to be free, but was resigned to having been sentenced to be blind for life with no chance of parole nor would she get time off for good behavior.

***

Jack Alvarez woke up with a splitting headache. He had gone to bed the previous night fully clothed after a bout with a bottle of tequila. Evidently, the bottle of tequila had won because the bottle was gone and the clock on the nightstand indicated he had less than an hour to get to his niece's birthday party. No time to shower, no time to shave, no time to buy a gift, but he had to be ontime or his sister would never forgive him. Seeing several Powerball Lottery tickets on the nightstand, he threw them in an empty box, wrapped the box in tissue paper, and taped a red bow left over from last Christmas on top. What the hell, his niece was blind—with any luck, she wouldn't be able to tell the difference. He quickly combed his hair, grabbed the gift, and exited out the door. Yes, his niece could rely on Uncle Jack. He would always be there when she needed him.

***

Lynda's mother announced the gift giver's name, then handed her daughter the gift. After Lynda opened the gift, Lynda would feel it all over, declare what she thought it was, and thank the giver. This worked well for all of the gifts until they came to the one from Uncle Jack:

"This box is empty," exclaimed Lynda as she handed it back to her mother.

"No, there is a gift card or something at the bottom," corrected her mother, turning the open box upside down. Out fell two thin cardboard rectangles. "Two lottery tickets. Knowing Jack as I do, they are most likely losers just like him. You know how the saying goes, 'birds of a feather flock together.' How could you do it to her, Jack! Isn't it enough that you are addicted to gambling? "*Perro*, now you are trying to infect *su sobrina* with your disease! How could you stoop so low? *Sin verguenza.*"

Jack had grown used to his older sister berating him for what she regarded as "his deficiencies." She wasn't Jack's mother and he would continue to live the lifestyle he had chosen no matter what his older sister thought of it. Still, it rankled him that she was trying to poison Lynda's mind against him.

Lynda's mother placed the two lottery tickets on an end table next to a phone and promptly forgot about them.

When Lynda's mother brought out the birthday cake with 23 lit candles, Lynda could feel the heat from the candles, but to her it looked like a big blur topped by a single flame.

***

A week later, Jack heard on television that a local liquor store which he frequented had sold the winning Powerball Lottery ticket to an unidentified customer. In checking the numbers, Jack found that both tickets were winners, one for the GRAND PRIZE and the other for $12,000.

Jack phoned Lynda's mother. Since Lynda had accompanied her mother on a shopping trip, there was no one at home to answer it. Jack shouted into his cellphone that Lynda had won the $585 million GRAND PRIZE plus $12,000 on the second ticket. "It turns out that the lottery tickets were no more losers than I am. Have a bitchin' nice day!," Uncle Jack summed up.

At first Lynda's mother refused to believe that Lynda's tickets had actually won more than a half billion dollars. She figured it was just another one of her brother's tricks. Once when they were children Jack had convinced her that a hollow tree in their backyard was full of bees. She still avoided that type of tree even though years ago she had discovered that Jack had been funning her. It was not until a local TV station confirmed that Lynda had won the Powerball Lottery that her mother quit suspecting that Jack was playing a cruel joke on them.

Lynda had several options for cashing in the winning tickets. She could take the money in monthly checks and avoid paying millions of dollars in taxes or she could take it all in one lump sum and let the Internal Revenue Service take a big (more like giant) bite out of it. Lynda chose the latter. When a morning talk show host asked her what she intended to do with the money, she said she was willing to give it all to any doctor or hospital that could cure her blindness. "Help me to see," she pleaded. "All I want is to escape the darkness which surrounds me 24 hours a day. Nothing is worth more than watching a sunrise over the Pacific Ocean or a hummingbird in flight. Give me that and you can have the rest." To emphasize her point, she broke the band on a stack of twenty dollar bills and tossed them in the air as she exited stage right, cane in hand.

***

Lynda was determined to do everything she could to restore her sight, especially now that she could afford the best doctors and the latest cutting-edge treatments. She started by making an appointment with a gene therapy clinic that sponsored a wellness program on a Sunday morning radio show. An ad for the Whyte Clinic claimed that researchers had achieved a major breakthrough in the treatment of inherited diseases. She figured she might as well give the Whyte Clinic a try. It was as good a place as any to start.

***

"Good afternoon," said the physician as he entered the exam room. "I'm Dr. Ostrowski," he continued, extending his hand in greeting. Then, seeing the white cane that was leaning against his patient's lap, he quickly withdrew it. "According to your chart, you are looking to restore your vision. The Whyte Clinic is currently conducting a study in which we are seeking to cure hereditary blindness by means of gene therapy and infusions of stem cells. Participation is voluntary. Since most insurance plans will not pay for treatment we offer a modest stipend to cover travel expenses. Would you like to take part in our study? It involves bi-weekly appointments over a six to nine month period.

"Of course, I would love to take part in the study," Lynda said, "I'm interested in doing anything that might restore my sight. How do I sign up?"

"Ask the Medical Assistant at the front desk for the necessary forms," Dr. Ostrowski advised. "You will also need to get a DNA throat swab, a blood test, and copies of your medical records for the past five years. You can speedup the process by having your medical files sent to the Whyte Clinic by Overnight Express. Any more questions? If not, then we can end this appointment. Have the girl at the front desk schedule an appointment for you to see me in two weeks."

Lynda had no sooner stepped out into the hallway when a loudspeaker blared, "CODE BLUE, CODE BLUE, ROOM A22!" She heard a medical cart rattling at high speed down the hallway and froze in her tracks. The medical technician pushing the crash cart attempted to swerve but clipped Lynda as he hurried by, sending her sprawling.

As Nurse Nit was responding to the Code Blue alarm, she saw Lynda fall. Ms. Nit helped Lynda stand up, examined Lynda for injuries, then led her into an exam room where Nurse Nit dressed minor lacerations to Lynda's left elbow. Because Lynda seemed disoriented, Nurse Nit had a doctor confirm that Lynda had not suffered any head trauma.

* * *

As part of the study, Lynda received gene therapy capsules along with massive macular injections of stem cells penetrating deep into the cornea. The injections were given at regular intervals, alternating between the right and left eye. The goal was for the influx of stem cells to replace dead or damaged cornea cells. It wasn't pretty, nor was it entirely without pain, but Lynda persevered and was rewarded with improved vision. So much so that at her 24th birthday party Lynda was able to see 19 of the 24 candles on her raspberry chocolate cake. She no longer used a cane to walk within the gated apartment complex. Following a minor dispute with the resident manager, Lynda purchased the apartment complex from the absentee owner, thus becoming her own landlord (plus that of the other tenants as well).

Shortly after Lynda's 24th birthday, the ocular study which had done so much to improve her vision was completed. During her final treatment, Lynda thanked Dr. Ostrowski for all he had done for her while reminding him that despite the improvement she was still legally blind. "Is there anything more that can be done?," Lynda asked.

"We have pretty much reached the current limits of gene therapy technology in North America. However, I will keep you posted as to any new developments," Dr. Ostrowski promised.

"You said we've reached the limits in North America. Does that mean that there are other countries that are ahead of us in gene therapy technology?," inquired Lynda. "Red Chinese researchers are pushing the envelope, mainly because they do not have the restrictions on human experimentation that our government imposes." Dr. Ostrowski confided. "Nonetheless, I doubt if they are that far ahead. If there had been any major breakthroughs, I most likely would have read about them in one of the medical journals that specialize in gene therapy. I do my best to keep abreast of what is happening in my field."

"Is there a chance that I could further increase my vision if I went to a Chinese medical institution that is conducting a trial similar to the one we are completing?" Lynda innocently asked.

"Of course, there is an outside chance," the physician confirmed, "but it would be a marginal chance at best. What is more likely is that they wouldn't be able to do anything for you at all or, much worse, they might cause you to lose some of the sight you recently regained. It's a crap shoot at best, but it is your decision to make. However, before you make up your mind, I think you should hear a story about something that occurred before either of us were born. Back in the early 1970's, during the Cold War, a distinguished Russian ophthalmologist developed a procedure called radial keratotomy to cure nearsightedness (myopia). Since it wasn't available in the United States, thousands of well-to-do Americans flew to Moscow to have the procedure done. So many Westerners came that the one hospital in which it was done instituted a factory-style surgical line in which a number of skilled surgeons each performed a separate incision in the complex corneal operation. In this way 40 to 50 operations could be done in one day. However, in the ensuing years unforeseen problems developed such as scar tissue and halo vision. As a consequence, today, radial keratotomy has been discredited. My colleagues and I have spent countless hours correcting the damage to sight that was done to thousands of Americans in Russia fifty years ago by an untested procedure. It's a shame that these over eager patients didn't have the patience to wait 10 years for U.S. ophthalmologists to develop and test laser surgery. To me, searching for "miracle" cures in foreign lands is largely a waste of time and money."

"Patience is the forbear of procrastination. To hesitate is the way to miss opportunities. I was in elementary school when I began to lose my sight," confided Lynda. "For fifteen years I put up with the darkness. It got me nowhere. Then your study came along and I began to see the light. If I wait, that light might vanish. As long as I have the resources to do so, I intend to pursue my goal of being able to see as good as anybody else."

"Understandable," responded Dr. Ostrowski since you

are bound and determined to go to China, I am going to give you the names of a few reliable Chinese researchers with whom I have had correspondence; that way you won't have to go in blind (please excuse the bad pun). At least you will have a starting point. *Bon voyage.*"

As Lynda was exiting the exam room, Dr. Ostrowski handed her a handwritten index card:

Yang Hui
Institute of Neuroscience
Shanghai, China

Institute of Vision Research
Yonsei University
Seoul, South Korea

***

Traveling to China for the first time would be a daunting task for any novice traveler, let alone for a blind person. Lynda felt she needed help. Rather than hire a stranger, she preferred to have Uncle Jack accompany her. After all, he had said that he would always be there when she needed him. The problem was that she had no way of knowing how long she would be staying in China. Lynda also needed someone to manage her apartment complex and other business affairs while she was away.

Who could assist her better than her own flesh and blood? But it did not seem fair for her to be continually asking them for help without any reciprocation on her part. No doubt it was time for Lynda to share her good fortune with her family.

Lynda broke the news to her mother and Uncle Jack that she would be going to China for an indefinite period of time when they were eating dinner at an Italian restaurant. She would be giving each of them five million dollars. They objected and said she didn't need to give them part of her winnings until she explained to them that they would be earning the money. Uncle Jack would be her chaperone/bodyguard during her stay in China and her mother would manage her investments at home.

In order to enter mainland China, Lynda and her Uncle Jack would need U.S. passports, tourist visas, and roundtrip airline tickets. Being inexperienced travelers, it took them six weeks to get everything in order.

They would be flying from Los Angeles International Airport (LAX) to Shanghai Pudong International Airport (PVG). Estimated non-stop flight flight time is 14 hours, 30 minutes.

Finally, the day of departure came. Lynda and her Uncle Jack left home two hours early to allow for possible delays at airport security. First rain, then hail began to fall. Being Southern Californians used to a relatively dry climate, neither Lynda nor Jack had thought to bring along a raincoat or an umbrella. No problem. The International terminal at Los Angeles Airport had more retail stores and kiosks than a shopping mall (and higher prices aimed at captive travelers). Jack had no trouble finding a shop that sold folding umbrellas. He bought two.

W hen Jack's luggage went through a metal detector, an alarm sounded. A Transportation Security Administration agent put the offending bag under a fluoroscope and all hell broke loose. Suddenly, Lynda and Jack were surrounded by TSA agents. A Los Angeles Airport policewoman pinned Jack to the ground while two TSA agents searched his pockets. They put handcuffs on Jack, then half-dragged, half-carried him to a small windowless room where they strip searched him, paying particular attention to his body cavities.

Meanwhile, Lynda was having difficulty finding someone who could tell her what was going on. She was panic stricken and started sobbing uncontrollably. A supervisor escorted Lynda to the room where Jack was being interrogated and explained that a fluoroscopy had revealed a nine millimeter Beretta in one of Jack's bags.

"Of course, he has a handgun. I hired him as my bodyguard. As you can see, I am blind. We are flying to China for ocular gene therapy that is unavailable in the United States. I don't know how long we will stay there," explained Lynda. "Frankly, I do not feel safe."

TSA agents fingerprinted Jack. They dumped the contents of Lynda's purse on a formica counter and confiscated her cellphone without giving her a reason. When a policewoman began to pat her down, Lynda said she would not cooperate further until she was allowed to speak to an attorney.

Forty minutes later two FBI agents, a man and a woman, arrived. After talking to the TSA people and reviewing the evidence they removed the handcuffs from Jack. No charges would be filed. Lynda and her Uncle Jack were free to board their flight to China. However, the handgun and a small bottle of cologne had been confiscated by the FBI agents. Lynda asked Jack why the agents objected to the cologne.

"Who knows? Who cares?", answered Uncle Jack. "We have five minutes to catch our flight. Let's go!"

Lynda and Jack were the last two people to board East China Airline's Flight 324 for Shanghai. Lynda's heart was pounding. She turned to Jack to make a comment, but Jack had fallen asleep after fastening his seatbelt. For Jack the gun incident had been nothing out of the ordinary. He lived on a gray edge between light and dark, good and bad. Such is the fate of the professional gambler. Little surprised him anymore. He took it all in stride. Uncle Jack wasn't completely jaded, but he was considerably more than halfway there.

Imagine spending fourteen and one-half hours on a non stop economy flight with no entertainment and cramped legroom. It's not the flight from hell, it's more like the flight from purgatory. One stewardess actually spoke passable English.

Pudong International Airport was not the inscrutable place that Lynda thought it would be. All signs were in both Mandarin and English. Also, there were money changing machines (dollar to yuan, etc.) in many areas of the International Terminal. However, Uncle Jack commented that they shouldn't be so fast to accept the exchange rate offered by the money changing machine. Jack had a hunch that the black market exchange rate would be more to their favor. Turns out, he was right. Soon after leaving the airport, they were approached by an English speaking Chinese gentleman in a business suit who offered to exchange their dollars for considerably more yuan than the money machine at the airport. It was a lesson in international finance that Lynda would put to good use in future travels.

Almost immediately Jack spotted a man in a leather jacket tailing them. He didn't seem to be too good at his job as he was following them at less than 10 feet. Jack was tempted to turn around and confront him, but since he was unarmed, he thought better of it.

Following a good night's sleep at a nearby hotel, Lynda and Jack took a taxi to the Institute of Neuroscience. Being home to more than 24 million people, Shanghai's streets were crowded. Traffic moved at a snail's pace. It seemed to take forever to get anywhere. What traffic lacked in speed, it made up with noise. Drivers shouting, horns honking, mixed with the sounds of new construction. And then there was Uncle Jack arguing with the taxicab driver over the fare. For Lynda, it was all too much. She shouted at Uncle Jack to pay the driver, she needed to get out. Her head was pounding from the sounds of the city. Surely, the esteemed Institute of Neuroscience could come up with two Tylenol tablets and a glass of water for a distressed damsel who had flown 6,500 miles to get there.

But it was not to be. In her miserable condition, she had difficulty making herself understood. Frustrated, Lynda left the Neuroscience Institute and lay down under a nearby tree. She sent Jack to buy a bottle of Tylenol. He returned an hour later to find Lynda sound asleep.

They spent the remainder of the day trying to find someone who was knowledgeable about the Neuroscience Institute's ongoing gene therapy research programs. Nobody seemed to know anything. Either that or the people they talked to were for an unknown reason being exceedingly tight-lipped. Jack thought it might be that since the Neuroscience Institute operated as a Chinese government facility, questions from information seeking foreigners were best left unanswered.

The man in a brown leather jacket with a bad haircut did not show up the second day. Jack doubted they would ever see him again. In the cloak and dagger world Lynda and Jack were small potatoes, hardly worth bothering with. When the initial surveillance proved fruitless, it probably was discontinued, Jack reasoned. The Chinese most likely had more important things to do than place a full-time tail on a couple of American tourists.

The Chinese economy was booming, posting double digit increases in most years. Each advance in technology brought with it a handful of new startups eager to exploit cutting edge research published by government funded institutions of higher learning. Most startups collapsed within two or three years, but the few who lasted generated immense profits for shareholders. Startups were constantly searching for "angel" investors who could overcome the initial financial inertia that new businesses inevitably encountered. However, Lynda was more interested in how a startup could improve her vision than she was with making money. She spent an entire day setting up appointments with gene therapy startups in Shanghai.

Lynda was surprised by what she found at the second startup she visited. The first startup had been exactly as she imagined - a small crowded office in a modern glass and steel high rise building headed by a Director who was more of a high pressure salesman than a businessman of substance and character. In her mind's picture of him there stood a sleazebag who would say or do anything to obtain one more cash fix. The second startup, Visual Sonar, Inc., located in a defunct cannery warehouse along the waterfront, smelled like a mixture of rotted fish and a dying diarrheic dragon's behind. However, what it lacked in style, it more than made up in substance. Its CEO pursued the novel idea of assisting sight with sound, much in the same way that a bat pinpoints the location of a mosquito on a moonless night.

Visual Sonar was already manufacturing a wristband with embedded sensors that alerted the wearer how close the nearest obstruction was by how long it took for a high-pitched sound to bounce of it and return. In fact, Lynda was so impressed that, following a tour of their assembly line and a look at Visual Sonar's financial records, she invested three million dollars in the business.

"You give him three million dollars and in return he gives you a plastic wristband worth $15," complained Jack as they left the former cannery. "Keep going at this rate and you will be broke inside of a year."

"Ever hear of Fitbit?," countered Lynda. "What Fitbit did for fitness buffs, this device, once it is properly developed, will do for sightless people. Besides, math was never your best subject. Spending money at the rate I have been going, it would take me more than a lifetime to go broke."

Their short-stay tourist visas were about to expire. A two week extension was granted to them. But the official who approved the extension was adamant that there would be no more extensions. If they wanted to stay in China longer than two more weeks, they would have to apply for a resident visa.

Being on a tight schedule and having nearly exhausted their prospects for ocular gene therapy in Shanghai, Lynda and her Uncle Jack decided to take a bullet train to Hong Kong where the City University of Hong Kong was said to be making great advances in gene therapy.

Traveling by bullet train proved to be a memorable, relaxing experience. Unlike on the jetliner, there was plenty of legroom. Not only was the scenery spectacular, the workers in the fields paused at their labor to wave at the train. Slightly more than eight hours after leaving Shanghai they arrived at West Kowloon Terminal in Hong Kong feeling refreshed, having slept for much of their journey.

Although Hong Kong was officially a part of China, in many ways it was a world apart. For one thing the local currency was the Hong Kong dollar rather than the yuan. Also, the general atmosphere seemed more open than in Shanghai where people were close-lipped, almost as if the Communist Party was monitoring every spoken or written word. Here, in Hong Kong, the street vendors and cab drivers were talkative, even on sensitive subjects such as government and religion.

In many ways Hong Kong has become the hyper-capitalist engine of commerce between East and West. Travel restrictions are in place to keep low-paid mainland Chinese from moving to Hong Kong which enjoys a higher standard of living.

Hong Kong became a colony of the British Empire after China ceded Hong Kong Island at the end of the First Opium War in 1842. The colony expanded to the Kowloon Peninsula in 1860 after the Second Opium War, and was further extended when Britain obtained a 99-year lease of the New Territories in 1898. The territory was returned to China in 1997. By treaty, Hong Kong maintains separate governing and economic systems until 2047 from that of mainland China under the principle of "one country, two systems," but in reality that principle is gradually being eroded by the Chinese government. It is only with constant vigilance that the residents enjoy such rights as they have. While the people of Hong Kong remain defiant, its administrators have a history of kowtowing to Chinese officials on issues in which the people of Hong Kong differ from their Communist masters.

Not having knowledge of the available lodging in Hong Kong, Lynda asked a taxicab driver to drive them to the nearest reasonably priced hotel. He took them to the Kowloon Grand Hotel which by its architecture and location was obviously a Western style luxury hotel, although in truth its $78 (USD) a night rate was reasonable by American standards, albeit extremely pricey by local norms.

Lynda screamed when she opened the door to her room on the 6th floor. Uncle Jack ran inside the room, expecting to tackle an intruder, but no one was there. Lynda explained, "I saw an enormous rat dash across the room and disappear into the far wall. We **need** to change rooms, pronto." Trying hard not to laugh, Jack told her that what her impaired vision took to be a rat was most likely a robotic vacuum cleaner. Still, to be on the safe side, he went back to the front desk and exchanged their rooms for two adjacent rooms on the 7th floor. The concierge took the incident seriously, knowing from experience that a rodent rumor could destroy business. He immediately apologized and arranged for an exterminator to check out the entire 6th floor for vermin.

The next morning, following a breakfast of rice sprinkled with grated dried mackerel and washed down with green tea, Lynda and her Uncle Jack went to Hong Kong City University. They did not have far to go as the university is located in the heart of Kowloon District.

The atmosphere at the university was completely different from that of academic institutions in Shanghai. Westerners comprised a significant part of the student body. Since most of the administrative staff spoke good English, Lynda had no trouble communicating to an administrative aide that she was seeking to become a subject in an ocular gene therapy research study.

After consulting her computer for several minutes, the administrative aide replied, "Yes, Professor Tan is currently enrolling subjects for a two year research study on cornea restoration. To apply you will have to fill out an application and return it along with a $!5 filing fee before the end of enrollment."

Lynda went back to her hotel room and with her Uncle Jack's help filled out the eight page application. Now, she was in the unenviable position of not knowing whether she would be accepted for the research study or how much longer she would remain in China.

Jack thought he could help her get the answers to her dilemma. Unbeknown to Lynda, Jack had been going down into the hotel basement for the past two nights to do some late night gambling with a few of the Kowloon Grand Hotel's off-duty laundry workers. They played Mah-Jongg with a $15 (Hong Kong dollars, HKD) limit. From the way they spoke, he figured they had a good knowledge of how to influence Hong Kong's administrative infrastructure. To hear them talk, it was (and had always been) blatantly corrupt.

At 2AM, the laundry room in the basement of the Kowloon Grand Hotel was oppressively warm and muggy. The acrid smell of stale beer and tobacco smoke hung in the air. A row of jumbo tumbling, whirring clothes dryers made it almost impossible for the four gamblers seated around a clothes folding table playing mah-jongg to hear each other. However, it did not deter Jack from attempting to start a conversation with the toothless man seated across the table from Jack, a red paisley bandana covering his head, looking very much like a 17th century pirate.

"Can't we turn on an air conditioner in here?" shouted

Jack, "it's stuffy in here!"

The wannabe pirate (or perhaps he was the real thing, Jack had no way of knowing) took a long drag off a stub of a cigar before responding, "No noisy air conditioner down here, and there is no need to yell, nobody here is hard of hearing."

"At least someone could open a window," Jack persisted.

"We are in the basement," the could-be, might-be pirate reminded Jack, "there are no windows. If you want to gamble in comfort, you can go across the bay to Macau, where you can pay big time for all the amenities your heart desires."

"You speak excellent English," stated Jack in an attempt to get on the man's good side.

"I was born in Hong Kong," explained the man Jack had mistook for a pirate, "although it may not be obvious at first glance, I am the product of an expensive English liberal arts education provided by our former colonial masters. Prior to independence, I was the head of the dockworker's union. My friends refer to me as 'Laoban'. The two other gentleman at our table are Jiang Zemin, former vice-president of the dockworker's union and Hu Jintao, former secretary of the dockworker's union." Jack nodded towards each man in turn as they were introduced to him. "As you can see, our political fortunes have severely declined since the departure of the British. Nevertheless, the current clamor for independence may place us back in power. *Shangdi tigong."*

"Shut up and throw the dice," exclaimed Hu Jintao.

Jack had no idea what the Chinese characters on the front of the tiles meant. Laoban said that "it does not matter because even an illiterate peasant can match the characters to win the game." Considering his losses at their last two sessions, Jack suspected otherwise.

Sure enough, Jack lost the game to Laoban. He had seen it before at a poker table in Gardena, California. Three friends schemed together to cheat a newcomer at cards. All three of the conspirators were from the same background.

Because he was a foreigner, this time Jack was the outsider. Being a professional gambler and having been fooled by conspirators before, Jack could kick himself for not seeing it coming. That time in Gardena, he and two friends had hid behind some dumpsters in the alley behind the poker casino waiting for the three cheaters to make their getaway. Jack did not have to wait for long. As the card sharks were piling into a car parked in the alley, Jack and his friends came out from behind the dumpsters and proceeded to smash the vehicle to smithereens with aluminum baseball bats.

That was 15 years ago. Jack had been younger and a whole lot meaner then. Also, there was three times as much money involved. Besides, Jack's primary purpose for being here was to gain information on how to influence Hong Kong's administrative decisions.

Putting aside the fact that he had been fleeced by amateurs, Jack decided to describe Lynda's dilemma straight up and seek Laoban's help with the matter while, having just won, Laoban was in a good mood.

"Contrary to what most foreigners believe, despite being nominally ruled by the Communist Party, Hong Kong is obsessed with materialism. Bribery is most effective when it is disguised as a donation," Laoban offered. "Money not only talks, it lubricates administrative decisions. American Vice-President Spiro Agnew was dismissed for having accepted $5,000 from a construction contractor for approving a multi-million dollar highway project. If the same thing had occurred in Hong Kong, Agnew-san would have lost face for being influenced by such a paltry amount."

***

"You need two things, a residency permit and inclusion in the cornea restoration research study headed by Dr. Tan, and you need to get both of them fast," Jack told his niece. "That means you need to expedite matters by bribing the officials in charge. Only you can't call it a bribe. Refer to it as a gratuity or a donation, whatever seems appropriate, as long as there is no connotation of corruption."

Lynda and her Uncle Jack were the first two people through the brass and glass double doors when the Hang Seng Bank opened at 10 AM. An older English speaking female bank teller performed a wire transfer from one of Lynda's banks in California, charging a 1.5 percent fee plus, as Jack suspected, converting U.S. dollars to Hong Kong dollars at the ridiculously low official exchange rate decreed by the mainland Chinese government. Lynda could have gotten a far better exchange rate on the Kowloon black market but she did not have time to shop around. Lynda stuffed $18,000 in hundred dollar bills into her purse and they left the bank, the entire transaction having been completed in less than 45 minutes.

Lynda hailed a taxi and instructed the driver to take her to the Hong Kong Public Security Bureau (PSB) Exit and Entry Administration office where she paid $140 to apply for a 10 year resident visa. While being interviewed by an official who would determine whether she qualified for a resident visa, she mentioned that she needed the new visa prior to becoming a subject in Dr. Tan's research study and was willing to pay extra for express service.

"Of course, we can process your application in a week for $500," the smiling official offered. "Should you be in a hurry, I can have your resident visa ready within an hour. To drop what we are doing, make the proper background checks, and have my boss sign off on it would cost $5,000."

Forcing a smile, Lynda removed five $1,000 banded bundles from her purse and placed them on the desk in front of the official. The balding administrator scooped up the money, asked to be excused, and left the room, closing the door behind him. In less than an hour, he returned, two resident visas in hand, one for Lynda and the other for her Uncle Jack. "A pleasure doing business with you," remarked the smiling official as he vigorously shook Lynda's hand. "If there are ever any complications, do not hesitate to contact me."

Street food sold by pushcart vendors in China's large cities is for the most part delicious plus it is inexpensive and convenient. For these reasons the Alvarez's ate most meals out, avoiding the excessive paperwork and expense of room service. However, Jack had purchased an electric combination vegetable steamer and rice cooker at Kowloon's marketplace; tonight would be one of the few occasions when they chose to "eat in." During dinner, Lynda remarked on how helpful the government official had been in expediting their resident visas.

"Money talks," ventured Jack. "My acquaintances tell me

everybody and everything has it price in Hong Kong. It's capitalism on steroids in an authoritarian society."

The only exceptions are handgun registrations and carry permits. Nobody other than the People's Liberation Army and the police are allowed to have weapons. I get the impression that the government doesn't trust its citizens with firearms, which is ironic considering that China invented gunpowder in the 10th century. Personally, I do not feel fully dressed without a handgun. No wonder the Chinese are so good at martial arts. A man needs to feel like he can protect his family should the situation warrant it."

Lynda awoke the next day to the sound of loud noises coming from the street below. Gazing out the window, Lynda saw colorful fireworks bursting in the air and what appeared to be a 30 foot dragon twisting from curb to curb as it sashayed its way through Kowloon accompanied by crowds of costumed revelers.

When she opened the door between their adjoining rooms for Jack, the first thing Lynda said was "What is going on out there?"

"Today is January 25, 2020, the first day of the Chinese Lunar New Year," explained Jack. "It's the year of the rat."

"Why would the Chinese celebrate twelve months rife with rodents?" Lynda wanted to know. "There is nothing funny about bubonic plague. We had to evacuate the 6th floor due to rats. I suppose now they are going to take over the entire hotel. Where is vector control when you need it? Quick, notify the World Health Organization."

"This is a cute stylized rat, the Chinese equivalent of Mickey Mouse," reasoned Jack.

"The rat I saw on the 6th floor looked mean," asserted

Lynda. "Filthy, probably diseased, definitely not anything Walt Disney would try to market."

"You could not tell a rat from a robot vacuum," stated Jack, "much less whether he looked cute or mean."

"Since we are going to be staying in Hong Kong for two years, we need to lease a house. Hotels are expensive. They cater to tourists, businessmen, and diplomats," concluded Lynda, "people on the move. Not for us. We need to blend in with the locals. Tomorrow, when I go to register at the university, I would like for you to see whatever passes for a real estate agency in this country. Rent a condominium or a house here in Kowloon. I want hot running water and a serviceable kitchen. A small garden would be nice."

***

Uncle Jack was right about how to get things done in Hong Kong. Facilitated by a $7,500 donation to the university's building fund, obtaining approval to take part in Dr. Tan's research study was fast and easy. Lynda was so impressed by the campus and the friendliness of the student body that she decided to enroll as a freshman.

When Lynda returned to the hotel, she found Uncle Jack in a foul mood. What did it to him were the ridiculously high rents in Kowloon.

"A two bedroom apartment rents for $2,500 a month, not including utilities and incidental fees," Jack wailed, "and that is with having to share a bathroom with the apartment next door. These real estate agents are pirates. I was lucky to escape the real estate agency with the gold fillings in my teeth intact."

" Don't fret," remarked Lynda, "I am pretty sure I have found a way around the housing problem that will also solve most of the other issues we are facing. If we enrolled as students, we could both live on campus for less than $600 a month, utilities included.

"Me a student?," Jack exclaimed. "I barely made it through high school. It's too late for me to get an education. Most likely I would embarrass you by flunking out. You go ahead. I can work as a stevedore on the docks while you are attending classes."

"You doing coolie labor? No way." Lynda reached out and latched onto her uncle's right hand. "Soft hands with no calluses. Physical labor is not your forte. I can hire you a tutor. What's the matter? It scares you, doesn't it?," guessed Lynda. "Look on the bright side, you will be surrounded by naive, gorgeous, young single females, some of whom will no doubt fall for your insipid, 'Hi, My name is Jack. I am an Aquarius, what's your sign?' pickup line. This is your time to shine."

"I'm phoning Mom and asking her to send us our high school transcripts," Lynda stated as she took her cellphone out of her pocket. "You did graduate, didn't you?"

"Of course I did," Jack replied, "East Los Angeles High, Class of '88. They taught me English and Spanish. The only thing I can say in Chinese is 'chop suey.'"

"Chop suey is as American as apple pie," corrected Lynda. "It was created in San Francisco by Chinese immigrants. I am not positive, but from what little I have heard most of the classes are taught in English. Besides, we could both benefit from learning to speak Chinese."

"Living on campus might have drawbacks," Jack speculated. "What if the bed is too hard? At home I have an orthopedic pillow top mattress."

"No, I won't spoil it for you," conceded Jack. "But I doubt if our class schedules will be identical, so how about if I get you a seeing eye dog to assist you when I am not around."

"I have been thinking about getting a service dog for quite some time," stated Lynda. "Let's look into it."

What Lynda and Jack found was that visually impaired people were using seeing eye dogs in China as early as the 13th century, long before the western world. However, it was not until 2012 that the Chinese government passed a law prohibiting public places from banning seeing eye dogs. Although the law has not been rigidly enforced, fewer public places are turning away service dogs.

Two days later, Lynda visited Hong Kong Seeing Eye Dog Services where she made a generous donation and started the process of obtaining a nine month old female black Labrador seeing eye dog named Lady Dei.

There were advantages to acquiring a service dog in China rather than in the United States. Service dogs are not required to be neutered in China and the cost of the dog and its training is most often less.

However, there would be a delay before Lay Dei could go home with Lynda. Lady Dei had two more months of seeing eye dog basic training to complete. Then there would be from one to two weeks of advanced training in which Lynda would participate as the two of them teamed up to confront the challenges which the visually impaired face on a daily basis.

Similar to the previous research study in which Lynda was a subject, Dr. Tan required her to have an injection in her cornea bi-weekly plus take several pills orally on a daily basis. The injections alternated between her left and right eyes. The shots were more scary than they were painful.

Classes started three week after Dr. Tan's ocular research study began. Both Lynda and Jack were listed as undeclared majors. Lynda took two classes in higher mathematics, a course in marketing, and a class in Basic Chinese. Jack took the same Basic Chinese class as Lynda. He also took a course in game theory and two classes in geology. Jack thought he was the oldest undergraduate student at the university. He wasn't. He simply had yet to encounter any students older than himself.

Learning what to do and what not to do to get along with the Chinese did not come easy. Jack liked to use his chopsticks as if they were drumsticks. He would tap out a rhythm on a tabletop, sometimes becoming totally involved. Chinese culture considered such behavior extremely rude. Also, he spit fishbones out into his rice bowl, a definite no-no. Whereas Lynda made friends easily, many students regarded Jack as a barbarian. Unlike Lynda, however, he kept his own company, seemingly unconcerned about what other people thought of him.

Bringing Lady Dei into the residence hall for the first time was a mixed experience. At first the residence hall's mother objected to having a dog inside the building, as did a few of the students. One made an official complaint. However, Hong Kong university's administrator for student housing ruled that assistance dogs were permitted by both university policy and Chinese law. An anonymous person slipped a note under Lynda's door at night which demanded that "the notorious flea and disease ridden beast" be evicted from the residence hall posthaste along with its "foreign devil" mistress. When

Lynda opened her hallway door the next morning she almost stepped in a pile of animal manure which someone had placed in front of the door.

That night Lynda showed Jack the "foreign devil" note and told him about the excrement in the hallway. Uncle Jack said the writer probably only sought to intimidate Lynda, but the phrase "foreign devil" led him to suspect there might be more to it. Later, when Jack went downstairs to gamble at Mah-Jongg, he related the earlier incident to the other three players. Laobahn took the matter seriously, commenting, "Your niece is in need of protection. Targeted people disappear. One day they are here, the next day they vanish, never to be heard from again."

Laobahn took out something wrapped in rags from an inner coat pocket and held it out towards Jack. When Jack went to take it with his right hand, Laobahn jerked it back, commenting that "Chinese etiquette demands that a person use both hands when accepting a gift."

Having been admonished, Jack used both hands to take the gift saying, "Whatever it is, it's certainly heavy."

"It's an 8 mm Nambu, together with a handful of bullets. There aren't many of them left," explained Laobahn when he saw the bewildered look on Jack's face. "The serial numbers have been filed off. Possessing an unauthorized firearm in China is a serious offense, even worse for a 'foreign devil.'"

Jack hefted the pistol in his right hand. "Please, allow me to pay you for it," Jack pleaded.

"You already have with your losses at Mah-Jongg," reasoned Leobahn. "Be careful. Government bugs and hidden cameras are everywhere in Hong Kong."

Now that Jack was packing a pistol, he felt he could better protect his niece from the Chinese hothead (Jack was relatively sure it was a Chinese student who had threatened Lynda, because seeing eye dogs were commonplace in most industrialized countries). However, he needed to fire the pistol to make sure it was in working order. On a day when there were no classes, he took the handgun along with two pillows to an unlocked shed and fired one shot into the ground, using the pillows to muffle the sound. Much to his surprise, the gun worked.

At the first reporting period, Lynda aced all of her classes. Unfortunately, Jack did nowhere near as well. Nevertheless, Lynda refused to give up on him. She hired a graduate student tutor to assist her uncle and insisted on weekly reports on Jack's progress. Following two weeks of tutoring, the tutor stated that "you can lead a horse to water, but you can't make him drink." Evidently, Jack wasn't motivated to learn and claimed to have an aversion to books.

Less than ten months into Dr. Tan's research study, something happened in another part of China which would have a profound effect on Lynda and her Uncle Jack. Biophysicist HE Jiankui announced that he and three colleagues had used CRISPR technology to modify human embryos and make them resistant to HIV, which led to the birth of twin girls, Lulu and Nana. The news immediately triggered worldwide criticism, denouncement, and debate over the scientific and ethical legitimacy of HE's genetic experiments. China's guidelines and regulations banned genome editing on human embryos for clinical use because of scientific and ethical concerns, in accordance with the international consensus. HE's human experimentation not only violated these Chinese regulations, but also breached other ethical and regulatory norms. These included questionable scientific value, unreasonable risk-benefit ratio, illegitimate ethics review, invalid informed consent, and regulatory misconduct. Intense international criticism led to HE being tried and convicted for practicing medicine without a license. The court sentenced HE to three years in prison and returned lesser sentences for his colleagues. Anxious to show its concern for moral and ethical issues, China's government chimed in by instituting a ban on all human gene editing experimental research.

Dr. Tan, his research team, and Hong Kong University were devastated. Lynda, whose sight was beginning to benefit from the biweekly treatments was heartbroken.

What to do? Dr. Tan's research study and all other Chinese CRISPR research studies involving human experimentation were suspended until further notice. It was clear to Lynda that China would no longer be on the cutting edge of treatment for Leber's congenital amaurosis. She was tempted to give up, pack her bags, and return to California. However, Jack and Lynda were enrolled in degree programs at Hong Kong City University. It would not make sense to simply pull up stakes and leave.

Later that night, Lynda told Jack about how the Chinese government had brought her ocular treatments to an abrupt halt. Jack's reaction was to suggest that they pack their bags and return to California as soon as possible. Lynda was against such precipitous behavior, but the only way she could get Jack to agree to stay until the end of the semester was to promise him an excursion to Macau, the former Portuguese colony that was rumored to have bigger and better casinos than Las Vegas.

In some ways student culture at Hong Kong City University resembled that of their counterparts in the western world. One way in which it did not, was in the Hong Kong

City University students' taste in foods. French fries, steaks, and hot dogs were rarely, if ever, part of their diet. One way in which it did was in western clothes (T-shirts, bluejeans, and tennis shoes). Jack had four yellow T-shirts silkscreened with the phrase "foreign devil" in red, bold block letters on the front of the T-shirt on the chance that it might provoke the person who had slipped the offensive note under Lynda's door to reveal himself. It didn't work. What did happen was that a number of students (several of whom were Chinese) began wearing "foreign devil" T-shirts. So much for Jack's investigative skills.

***

On their next two days without classes, Lynda and her Uncle Jack took a ferry from Hong Kong to Macau, a distance of about 41 miles. Everything they had heard about Macau turned out to be true. Macau has 38 casinos and it takes in more revenue from gambling than Las Vegas. Jack stood in awe of its glitz and glamor, but was disappointed when he discovered that the free drinks being passed out by lovely hostesses consisted of various varieties of tea. Unlike Reno and Las Vegas, alcoholic drinks did not flow freely.

They took two adjoining rooms at the Grand Lisboa Palace for one night at a cost of less than $200. The word 'palace' was not a misnomer. It was truly palatial with gold bathroom fixtures and canopy beds. Nor did the management attempt to prohibit Lady Dei from staying in Lynda's room.

Lynda took advantage of the hotel's indoor spa while Jack went down to the casino to gamble. The majority of the games were of western origin. There was only one that Jack did not readily recognize. At 3 AM Lynda heard Jack enter his room. From the racket emanating from his room, he had more to drink than the free tea. Lynda rolled over and went back to sleep.

Despite Lynda's efforts to wake up Jack, he did not get up the next day until almost noon. Even then, he looked like shit, but Lynda avoided commenting on it.

That night, they took the ferry back to Hong Kong. Since the bay was choppy and Jack had yet to recover from the previous night's revelry, he spent a lot of time leaning over the railing. Lynda left him alone so as not to embarrass him.

Student life had paled for Lynda with the abrupt end of Dr. Tan's research study. Her hopes had gone sky high only to be dashed against the immovable rock that was the omnipresent, authoritarian Chinese government. Lady Dei was the bright spot in Lynda's life. Hugging Lady Dei helped Lynda deal with depression.

Jack struggled to do better in his classes. His problem was that his heart was not into studying. He seized upon the slightest distraction as an excuse to set aside his books. It bothered him that his niece put such a heavy emphasis on his education. After all, he was nearing middle age and was set in his ways.

Lynda heard from a teaching assistant that Dr. Tan had gone to South Korea where he was able to restart his research study. She was tempted to follow, but thought better of it. She had gained little of the visual improvement she had hoped to get by traveling to China and there was no reason to believe that traveling to South Korea would turn out any better. In fact, she regretted having gone abroad to seek treatment. Dr. Ostrowski had warned her of the dangers of traveling abroad for treatment, but Lynda had rejected his advice.

Lynda and her Uncle Jack started making plans for going back to the United States. There would not be much to pack. Much of their non-essential items had already been sent to Lynda's mother for safekeeping.

It was not as if traveling to China had been a complete waste. Lynda now owned a near majority of shares in a startup which manufactured sonar wristband distance finders for visually challenged individuals such as herself. Administrative officials assured Lynda that all class credits for her freshman year at Hong Kong City University would be accepted by the University of California, Irvine, towards earning a degree. And, best of all, Lady Dei and Lynda had become inseparable, each dependent on the other. Her Introductory Biology professor referred to the relationship between Lynda and Lady Dei as a perfect example of "symbiosis." Nor was a service dog acquired in China required to be spayed as they were in the United States, often leading to listlessness, obesity, and a significantly shortened lifespan.

The semester was drawing to an end. High time to pay attention to the details of Lynda and Jack's return to California.

Hampering their progress, was the Chinese government's knee jerk response to an attempted hijacking of a jetliner a week earlier. Although nobody was injured or killed and the bad guys with the fake bomb were all Chinese dissidents, security was immediately tightened and foreigners were rounded up and interrogated in an attempt to expose it as a CIA plot.

Two plain clothes detectives who spoke perfect English had approached Jack as he was headed off campus and herded him into the backseat of a late model sedan driven by a Hong Kong police officer who drove them to a nearby police station. Jack was frisked, but the detectives did not place him in handcuffs. After an hour of interrogating Jack in a windowless concrete block room that stunk of sweat and stale tobacco smoke, a uniformed Hong Kong police officer drove him around in what seemed to be steadily increasing ellipse before dropping Jack off on a wide sidewalk facing the campus. No charges were brought against him.

This was not the first time Jack had been interrogated. Anytime anything goes wrong in China, the national impulse is to find a foreigner to blame it on. Taken as a whole, Chinese culture is xenophobic. However, Jack found it understandably so. In the 19th century, European powers tried to carve up China, worse yet, they largely succeeded. What followed was the First and Second Opium Wars, the Boxer Rebellion, and the siege of Manchuria; all of which China (then known as the Celestial Kingdom) lost.

Jack had discovered first hand through his relations with former Hong Kong dockworkers that it was not enough to be Chinese or of Chinese heritage. To be fully accepted, one had to be Han Chinese. Uighurs and other ethnic groupings are largely excluded. Jack had no trouble understanding this, either, because the United States had recently undergone a long period of Isolationism and still struggled with racial issues. Understanding a problem is one thing, going along with it is quite another. As Jack had been telling Lynda for months, "the sooner we leave China, the better."

* * *

Finally, the day (or to be proper, night) of departure arrived. The semester was over, grades had been posted, and Jack had actually earned an "A" in Biology. Lynda and her Uncle Jack would be departing Hong Kong on a non-stop redeye Air China flight to Los Angeles. This time they knew to bring plenty of reading material and several hand held video games with them. Surprise of surprises! Lady Dei was allowed to accompany Lynda in the cabin at no extra cost, with the provision that she wore a muzzle and remained on a leash at all times.

There had been good moments during their extended stay in China, and Lynda and Jack had both gained knowledge at the City of Hong Kong university. Overall, their trip had been a rewarding experience (despite the fact that Jack would have felt much more comfortable if he had stayed home in California). Jack's 8 millimeter pistol remained behind, buried beneath the floor of a seldom used shed on the outskirts of the City of Hong Kong university. In Jack's mind, it was his gift to some future human-rights-and-freedom-loving generation of Chinese. *May it soon come to pass.*

CHAPTER 4

The Selkirk family had been farming in rural Ontario, Canada, for more than 150 years. The current patriarch, Big John Selkirk, 6 foot 3 inches and 200 pounds of solid muscle in Oshkosh overalls and a Toronto Blue Jays baseball cap, took pleasure in emphasizing how unforeseen circumstances and the vagaries of a short growing season had made the Selkirks tough and self-reliant. Two or three good years were often followed by a string of lean years. Family farming was a hard way to make a living. Workdays started at sunup and rarely ended before sundown.

Despite extensive use of pesticide, European cornborers destroyed twenty percent of the Selkirk family's cash corn crop in the previous growing season. That meant that they suffered a net loss. The Selkirk's could survive operating in the red for one year, but if it happened two years in a row, they would be in serious financial trouble.

In late Fall, Big John was sitting on the front porch of their two-story farmhouse, debating whether or not to plant corn in the upcoming summer season, when two middle-aged men in a dusty late model 4-door Ford sedan pulled up to the house. Before the men stepped out of their car, Big John had already guessed by their change-of-clothes hanging from wire coat hangers suspended from a nearly rolled-up rear window that they were traveling salesmen, or 'damn drummers' as his great-grandfather used to call them.

"Whatcha selling?," derisively greeted Big John, not bothering to rise from his chair as the salesmen slowly mounted the five concrete steps that led up to the porch.

"Good afternoon, Mr. Selkirk. I'm Jeff and this is my partner, Ron," replied Jeff, ignoring Big John's less than friendly welcome as the two salesmen sat in wooden chairs on the large wooden porch opposite Big John. "We represent Monsanto, the company from whom you bought a substantial amount of Bt pesticide last season. Judging from my conversation with other farmers in this area, the European corn-borer nearly destroyed last year's corn crop, even for those farmers like yourself who applied the maximum amount of pesticide allowed by law. That tiny, moth-like one inch long insect is rapidly becoming resistant to what we sold you. Monsanto is taking full responsibility for any losses you suffered. Our scientists have developed Bt corn, a perfectly safe variety for humans that is lethal to corn-borers. We want to regain your trust in our products, so we are going to supply you with your first year's supply of Bt seed corn absolutely free. That's right, gratis, at no cost to you. Our researchers estimate that Bt corn will yield you a 50 percent greater harvest than the corn you have been planting. Mind you, that's a conservative estimate. So, how about it? Can we strike a deal?," Jeff asked as he stood, smiled, and extended his right hand toward Big John.

Big John was in no mood for either a smile or a handshake. Swiveling in his seat until he was looking Ron in the eyes, he stood and said softly, "We need to go in the house, sit down at the kitchen table, and discuss this further."

***

"What is Bt? It seems that the products you guys sell are Bt this, and Bt that. Fill in the letters between 'B' and 't' and you get 'Bullshit', which is what Monsanto sold me last year. I must look like a rube to you. Why else would you be pulling this Bt scam two years in a row?," Big John asked with furrowed brow while struggling to control the anger rising inside him.

"Let's start with the technical definition," Ron suggested. "After that we can dig into what it means for Monsanto and what it can do for you. **Bt** (*Bacillus thuringiensis*) is a bacterium found in soils throughout the world. It naturally produces crystal-like proteins (Cry proteins) that selectively kill a few specific insect species. Bt corn, also known as transgenic corn, is corn that has been genetically modified to produce the insecticidal proteins that occur naturally in Bt. Monsanto originally made use of Bt by spraying it on crops to kill insects. That, as you well know, had mixed results. Then, one of our bright researchers came up with the idea of adding Bt to the corn itself. It seems that Bt has no effect on humans, but it is curtains for the pupal stage of the European corn-borer. Our test results are an 80 percent kill rate for Bt when used as a pesticide and a 99 percent kill rate when Bt becomes an integral part of the corn itself."

"Monsanto now acknowledges that Bt is only partially effective when used as a pesticide. We didn't mean to screw you," Jeff apologized. "In order to remain in business Monsanto requires the goodwill of farmers like yourself. Like I said earlier, we are going to give you the first year's Bt seed corn for free. Not only that, Monsanto will also buy your entire first harvest of Bt corn for 15 cents per bushel above current market value. There you have it—guaranteed success. It's a deal that will make you the envy of every farmer in North America."

"I've always supplied my own seed corn from last year's harvest just as farmers have been doing for thousands of years. Now you come along and offer me one year's supply of Bt seed corn for free. It sounds insane, but common sense tells me that Monsanto didn't become the giant that it is by giving away the store. There must be a method to your madness," Big John reasoned. Could it be that Bt corn is a sterile hybrid in the same way that a mule is the sterile hybrid offspring of a horse mating a donkey? Or is it like heroin: the first time is free. Then, once you are hooked, the dealer forces you to turn your pockets inside out. And if that isn't enough, he flips you upside down and shakes you until he is satisfied that he has taken your last penny."

"That's a horrible analogy," exclaimed Jeff. We're legitimate businessmen, not heartless criminals. If you can get a better deal elsewhere, do so."

"What puzzles me is why a giant U.S. corporation would seek out an isolated Canadian dirt farmer like myself? You two are a long way from home. That makes sense. A dog doesn't want to shit in his own backyard. Does Monsanto think it would be easier to cover up it's corporate shit out here in rural Ontario than it would be if they tried to do it in the United States?," Big John considered.

"You are right about Monsanto singling you out because you are remote, but it is not about covering up. Monsanto is concerned that Bt corn pollen might negatively affect nearby crops. Your nearest farming neighbor is more than a kilometer away. Yes, we want to use you as our guinea pig. However, you will be the happiest guinea pig of all with a wallet fat enough to choke a horse," Ron confessed. "An opportunity like this doesn't happen every day. Seize it while you can."

"I will mull it over," equivocated Big John while pretending to suppress a yawn. "Of course, I would think a lot more about it if Monsanto guaranteed me 25 cents per bushel above market value for two years and agreed to grant me a $2,400 loan at two percent interest, so I can repair the harvester."

"You drive a hard bargain," concluded Ron as he stood up from the table and turned towards the front door. "I will phone the head office first thing tomorrow and see if they will go along with it. I'm fairly sure they will accept your terms.

For the next two years, Big John Selkirk planted Bt corn and got spectacular results. Bt corn grew 6 inches taller, had 10 percent more ears, and yielded 28 percent more bushels than standard varieties.

Unbeknownst to the salesmen, Monsanto researchers had recently added a "super sweet" gene to the Bt corn genome. It was the "super sweet" taste that endeared Bt corn to the public.

After the first year's harvest, Big John bought a new candy apple red F-150 Ford truck and paid off the $2,400 loan from Monsanto.

Following the second year's harvest, Big John renovated his aging farmhouse and built a new barn. Currently, he is planning on taking his family on an extended ocean cruise to the South Sea islands. Most surprisingly of all, Big John trashed his Toronto Blue Jays baseball cap. He now wears a lime green broad brim baseball cap with a red and white "Big M" Monsanto logo emblazoned on the front that was given to him by Ron and Jeff in appreciation of the good things he said about them in an interview published in a recent edition of Modern Canadian Agriculture magazine.

Last year, when the Royal Bank of Canada foreclosed on the delinquent mortgage of a nearby farm and the mortgagor moved to Toronto, the Selkirks looked into buying it from the bank, but the bank wanted to sell it at market value, which was well above the amount that Big John offered. After the farm sat vacant for a year, however, the Royal Bank of Canada decided to accept the Selkirk's original bid. As soon as the farm clears escrow, Big John is planning to double the acreage he devotes to Bt corn. Ontario has become an exporter of Bt corn to ethanol plants in the United States. As Big John likes to put it, "good things happen to good people."

CHAPTER 5

Antara Biswas was born in Bihar, one of the poorest provinces in India. Her father, Anil, inherited a .23 acre plot of agricultural land from his recently deceased father on which he tried to grow enough rice to feed his family.

Less than one-quarter acre of prime farmland would not be considered worth farming in most nations, much less the worn out soil that the Biswas family had tilled for as long as anyone could remember. Fortunately, Anil's older brother who had inherited the lion's share of the family farm was able to help out when food supplies ran low, but that was hardly a permanent solution since his brother had a wife, six children, and a mother-in-law to feed.

Anil's aging hand tools consisted of two hoes, a long pointed stick for planting seeds, and a rusted spade. What he wanted most was a water buffalo. Surely, Lord Krishna, having in the beginning been a villager himself, would answer his faithful servant's prayers by providing one.

Antara was small for her age. A routine school medical checkup discovered a severe rash on her chest and minor vision problems. The healthcare worker who interpreted the results suspected Antara was suffering from Vitamin A Deficiency (VAD), a condition which afflicts 11 percent of children, age 1 through 8 in India, largely the result of a diet consisting mainly of milled white rice.

A World Health Organization agent (WHO) persuaded Anil to forego white rice by offering Anil free golden rice seedlings a month before the monsoon rains came. Golden rice is white rice that has been genetically enhanced with a beta-carotene gene to provide Vitamin A.

Antara's body rash disappeared several months after Anil's first golden rice harvest and her sight began to get better shortly after that. Today her schoolwork has vastly improved as it has for thousands of India's schoolchildren who suffered from VAD.

Golden rice has been somewhat of a disappointment since it was first introduced to India in 1994 when it was touted as a panacea for India's many agricultural problems. It did not result in increased harvests and golden rice cost millions of dollars to implement. Nevertheless, it has been a life saver for millions of children with VAD globally. Golden rice has been both an economic failure and a health success. Antara and her father, Anil, say golden rice is worthwhile. A handful of bankers and politicians think otherwise. Ultimately, the public will decide the fate of golden rice.

PART II

CRISPR Horror

CHAPTER 6

Akari Seto and her younger brother, Haruchi, were latchkey children. Most mornings, following a breakfast of leftover rice and green tea, they walked to school and their parents boarded a company bus headed for the Hitatchi electronics factory on the outskirts of Tokyo where Mrs. Seto worked on an assembly line and Mr. Seto loaded trucks on the back dock.

Akari and Haruchi went directly to their family's second story apartment when school let out in the early afternoon. Since it would be hours before their parents returned home from work, they hurriedly did their homework and household chores, after which they sat cross-legged on the floor in front of a television set watching heroic animes, old Godzilla flicks, and repeats of NHK public television shows.

Akari enjoyed watching vintage Japanese black and white monster films, but Haruchi was obsessed with them. At night, he fantasized that he lived on Monster Island with Godzilla, Rodan, Mothra, Mechagodzilla, and a host of lesser-known creepy creatures from Japanese mythology.

Haruchi idolized Godzilla special effects artist, Eiji Tsuburaya, the man responsible for creating a miniature Tokyo set and having a man in a rubber suit play Godzilla. He even took to wearing a plaid hat that resembled the hat regularly worn by Eiji Tsuburaya.

Eventually, Akari outgrew her fascination with Japanese monsters, but not so Haruchi. He taped scary monster movie posters from Toho Productions to his bedroom walls along with a map of Monster Island.

For everyone, a time comes when childhood is over. We put away our playthings and become responsible adults. Akari became an Emergency Room Registered Nurse. Haruchi's fascination with sea monsters led him to become a research technician mapping genomes of commercial species of fish at an Osaka University oceanography lab. It was not unusual for Haruchi to bring his work home with him. What began as a desktop computer and a microscope in a corner of a spare bedroom soon grew into a personal well equipped genetics lab bench. Nor did he confine his efforts to editing the DNA of commercial species of fish.

One night, seemingly by accident, Haruchi wandered onto the dark web. After seeing videos detailing the results of various unauthorized genetic experiments, he came up with the idea of creating a real life, flesh-and-blood Godzilla. He began by buying a newly hatched male saltwater crocodile from an Australian man whose online identity was Reptile Ron. Three weeks later, he located a man on Mindinao who had a juvenile female kimono dragon for sale, but the man wanted $2,100 for it. Too much! However, following intense financial discussions via cellphone, Haruchi was able to get the price down to $625 plus a dozen glass slides of infectious bacteria.

Harachi knew that as a general rule, in order for two different species to successfully mate and produce hybrid offspring the progenitors must be mature and share approximately 95 percent of their genomes in common. That meant that he would have to wait for two years before he could perform an in vitro fertilization. Feeding and taking care of two large reptiles without anybody suspecting what he was doing was extremely difficult, but Harachi managed to do it. He also criss-crossed the dark web searching for samples of DNA scraped from the fossils of Tasmanian marsupial tigers, sabre-toothed tigers, ichthyosaur, Gigantopithecus, Megaladon, Mosasaurus, blue whale, and Tyrannosaurus Rex. In an attempt to give his Godzilla greater intelligence he also took samples from his own DNA and, unbeknown to her, a hair sample taken from his sister, Akari.

Everything had to be done in secret. Much of what he was doing was considered by the public to be unethical or immoral. Mixing animal and human DNA was illegal, nor was it legal for Haruchi to clandestinely obtain a sample of Akari's DNA.

Thirty-two months into his Godzilla Project, Harachi harvested four eggs from the kimono dragon and a small vial of sperm from the saltwater crocodile. After freezing three of the eggs and two-thirds of the sperm in a liquid nitrogen storage container, Harachi proceeded to combine the remaining egg with the remainder of the sperm in a petri dish. The resulting zygote divided rapidly over the next few days developing into four prototype Thunder Lizard embryos whose DNA would be painstakingly edited to produce four living, roaring, earth-shaking monstrosities, the likes of which had heretofore only been imagined in artsy horror flicks. As Pablo Picasso said, "We all know that Art is not truth. Art is a lie that makes us realize truth at least the truth that is given us to understand." And that is that. Otherwise, one is forced to acknowledge that Oscar Wilde had it right when he wrote in an essay that "Life imitates Art far more than Art imitates Life." In either case, Haruchi was destined to realize the prophetic vision of Eiji Tsuburaya.

The three Godzillas grew rapidly. Soon it became obvious that it was impossible to restrain them. Haruchi paid a welder to build three steel cages which could hold them until they could be released into the Sea of Japan.

Haruchi also leased a fishing boat. His plan was to release the triplet Godzillas off Sarushima Island in Tokyo Bay, but, not being much of a sailor, a storm came up and he got blown off course. He soon sighted land which he mistook for Sarashima Island. But in actuality it was Uotsuri-shima, the largest of the Senkaku Islands that are claimed by both China and Japan.

Shortly after anchoring off the coast of Uoturi-shima, one of the two crewmen whom Haruchi had hired to help him, spotted a Chinese patrol boat approaching them from a distance. The trawler's crew struggled to unlock the cages and release the three Godzillas into the ocean before the patrol boat could come into hailing distance. They were in such a rush that they inadvertently tipped one of the cages over the railing and into the ocean before unlocking it. The other two Godzillas jumped through the open cage doors into the sea when the Chinese patrol boat pulled alongside the fishing boat and secured it with grappling hooks.

The officer-in-charge of the patrol boat demanded to see their sailing documents. Since the Japanese vessel had no papers nor any fish in its hold, the Chinese officer became suspicious of Haruchi's intentions and arrested all three Japanese for violating Chinese territorial waters. The leased fishing boat was confiscated and towed to China where all three Japanese were interrogated and later tried for espionage. Despite the best efforts of the

Japanese Embassy, Haruchi was sentenced to 25 years in a communist labor camp near the border with Laos.

Haruchi had no way of knowing what happened to the triplet Godzillas following his arrest. He assumed the one who had gone overboard in a locked cage had perished. Perhaps the other two had fallen victim to a whale or a giant squid. Nothing could be farther from the truth. The first Godzilla had kicked apart his locked cage long before it reached the ocean floor. The other two joined him. Working as a team, they rid nearby waters of all predators other than themselves. When the Chinese patrol boat returned to Uoturi-shima six months later, they turned the boat into splinters and marooned its crew on Chiwei Island without food or water. Fortunately, they were rescued by a Nationalist Chinese submarine two nights after being stranded. They had slept on a pebble beach and ate mussels pried from rocks in shallow waters along the coast.

Gradually, the triplet Godzillas ventured further afield in search of prey. The first time that the media caught wind of them was when they came ashore at night at Hiroshima on August 6 during the floating lanterns peace ceremonies. Fifty thousand people witnessed their arrival first hand and the media broadcast pictures of the three Godzillas around the world. They left almost as quickly as they came, causing no damage according the *Japan Times* which published a lengthy editorial suggesting that the appearance of three Thunder Lizards at the Hiroshima Peace ceremonies was a thrice fortuitous omen foreshadowing good things to come.

Although the three Godzillas were identical triplets, closeup examinations of newspaper photographs revealed that they had differing birthmarks that permitted onlookers to tell them apart. The media labeled them Ichi, Ni, and San. Purportedly, they were brothers, Ni being the leader.

Increasingly, the triplet Godzillas followed the Japanese Current and other ocean gyres in search of more food to satisfy their ravenous appetites. In less than a year, they ate their way across the Pacific Ocean, approaching shore near the Port of Los Angeles, California, where an independent photographer shot a twenty-one minute video of the three siblings acting as a team in attacking a great white shark which they subsequently devoured. The video instantly went viral, having been watched by more than seventeen million people within one hour after having been posted online.

Ichi, Ni, and San came ashore at twilight near the Aquarium of the Pacific. Although it was closed, Ni smashed through a wall. Once inside, they were confronted with a number of giant tanks imprisoning a variety of sea creatures resembling those that the triplet Godzillas had encountered as they made their way across the Pacific Ocean. Suddenly, a thunderous alarm sounded and bright security floodlights flashed on. Startled, Ni smashed against a humongous, thick pane of glass, releasing thousands of gallons of seawater along with all sorts of sea life.

Angered, Ichi and San shattered tank after tank, flooding the enormous building that housed the Aquarium. Their appetites whetted by fish flopping about on the floor, the siblings stuffed themselves until they could hold no more. For the triplets, the Aquarium of the Pacific was like a pot of gold at the end of a rainbow; an all-you-can-eat supply of live sushi that provided a dining experience that only three ravenous Thunder Lizards could fully appreciate.

As the sun came up over the horizon, they trod north toward Los Angeles, leaving a wide swath of destruction in their wake. Bridges fell, freeway overpasses pancaked, buses overturned, and big rig trailers spilled their loads in a scene reminiscent of the 1971 Sylmar earthquake in which 24 people died. Roadblocks set up by the local police proved ineffective, the three Godzillas pushed them aside as if they were made of cardboard.

Several hours later, Ni smashed through the sliding glass entrance to the International Terminal at Los Angeles International Airport, San and Ichi following close behind. People panicked, screaming as they strived to put as much distance between themselves and the monsters as possible.

National Guard troops set up concrete barriers around the perimeter of the terminal. While under fire from troops huddling behind the barriers, all three Godzillas easily jumped over the barriers and ran onto a runway. Two Huey Cobra helicopters strafed the monsters with.50 caliber gatling guns. One helicopter came in low and Ichi swatted it out of the sky with a swing of his tail.

Residents of a nearby hotel watched in horror from their balconies as Ni and San tore down the air control tower while Ichi ravaged the hangers. A stray tracer bullet fired by a National Guard corporal penetrated a tanker truck full of J-4 jet fuel triggering an explosion which could be heard miles away in Gardena.

Continuing northward, the Godzilla triplets tromped their way through Beverly Hills, pausing at intervals to tear down wrought iron gates and cavort in Olympic size pools. Television camera crews filmed every destructive move. Via internet their feed was being streamed live to a global audience estimated at more than two billion viewers. Ni, Ichi, and San had become instant celebrities.

Drones flying overhead kept track of the monsters as they continued on their way northward. Two Hellfire missiles were fired at Ni by remote control operators. One went too high and exploded against an abandoned fire lookout tower. The second missile struck the ground inches behind Ni, but was a dud and failed to explode. Nonetheless Ni suffered a slight sprain to his left ankle which only served to increase his anger.

Ichi tore an ancient gnarled oak tree from the ground roots and all and hurled it at a ranger station, crushing two jeeps parked in front of the station. Fortunately, no one was injured.

Having reached the summit of the coastal hills, there was no other way to go but down. Because the backside of the coastal was steeper than the frontside there were no trails leading down into the valley below. That hardly deterred Ni. Lifting his enormous tail high in the air, he sat on his rump and slid over 500 feet down to the bottom of the hill, raising a cloud of dust and debris that made him sneeze which overturned a bus full of tourists that had just come to a full stop 25 feet away in the rear of a Universal Studios parking lot. Ichi and San followed.

Standing up, the three siblings thrashed their way toward a line of M1A2 Abrams tanks that were preparing to fire a volley of 120 millimeter depleted uranium shells at the monsters. The first volley whizzed overhead, missing the three brothers by mere inches. Before the tanks could load and fire a second round of projectiles, the Godzillas turned around and began running backwards toward the line of tanks, their tails held high, waving rapidly back and forth like gigantic windshield wipers. The triplet Godzillas had covered over half the distance to the line of tanks, when the tank crews fired their second volley.

This time the 120 millimeter projectiles were deflected by the monsters' heavily armored tails, cratering the asphalt parking lot. Before the tanks could reload and fire a third volley, the monsters were upon them tossing the 70 ton tanks in the air as if they were tennis balls. Growing tired of the sport, the siblings went through the arched entrance to the amusement park, racing forward at full speed through the upper lot and sliding down an escalator to the lower lot where the Godzilla triplets defeated and disassembled a platoon of mechanical Transformers, crushing them into metal blocks ready to be recycled at the scrapyard. All hail the dominion of living, breathing, reasoning lifeforms over battery powered mechanical robots which depend on artificial intelligence for guidance.

Looking up, Ni saw a large flock of seagulls circling overhead, soaring on warm air currents whenever possible. At the same time, Ni caught a whiff of sea breeze from the southwest, reminding him that it was time for the Godzillas to return to the Pacific Ocean where a sustainable life awaited them. Executing a 220 degree turn, Ni bypassed the regrouped Abram tanks, leading his brothers back into the coastal hills where they were harassed all through the night by assault helicopters and a mixed squadron of F-22, F-35 and Japanese F-3 jet fighters. It was like being attacked by a determined swarm of bees, annoying but by no means catastrophic.

As the sun came up in the East, the Godzilla triplets were tearing through the community of Westwood, ripping two-story houses from their foundations and throwing them at attacking helicopters. San jumped up from the roof of a high-rise building and snared an F-35 fighter, dashing it to the pavement below where it exploded in a tremendous ball of fire. Ichi urinated on it, dousing the flames.

Santa Monica and the Pacific Ocean loomed ahead. Ichi stomped apart Santa Monica Pier, upturning the ferris wheel and tossing it like a frisbee out into the breakers. Spotting a pod of gray whales cavorting in Santa Monica Bay, Ni, Ichi, and San waded into the ocean. A passing U.S. Navy guided missile cruiser fired upon the triplets. Ichi grabbed a shark and threw it at the cruiser, striking a boatswain in the chest as he stood near the bridge and sending him tumbling into the ocean where he was never seen again.

Wading out into the Pacific Ocean along the continental shelf, the Godzilla triplets permitted the California Current to sweep them along to where it joined the North Pacific gyre (much like the Missouri River flows into the Mississippi River) which they followed back to the Sea of Japan. Along the way, the Godzilla trio savaged a 41 foot Giant Squid, first stripping it of its eight tentacles, then devouring its great bulbous head. For 36 hours they feasted on Calamari Sashimi, a delicacy by Japanese standards. Leaving the leftovers to vicious shark scavengers, the satiated siblings went with the flow of the Japanese Current back to the Sea of Japan. Circling Uoturi-shima in search of their creator they found the formerly uninhabited island had significantly changed. While they were gone, the Japanese government had constructed a lighthouse and a wharf on the western tip of Uoturi-shima. Ichi waded ashore at midnight, intent on pulling down the towering bright light, but Ni intervened with a reverberating roar and stopped him. The Godzilla triplets had returned to their ancestral home.

There would be no more unwarranted destruction.

In a prisoner exchange, China released Haruchi to Japanese authorities. He had served four years of a 25 year sentence. He was given a hero's welcome home. Shortly thereafter, the Japanese Diet (legislature) overwhelmingly passed a bill designating the Senkaku Islands as a national park with severely restricted access and appointing Haruchi Seto as Chief Director of the Senkaku Islands and Lighthouse Keeper on Uoturi-shima. Haruchi is still obsessed with kaiju and the Godzilla triplets are respectful of their creator. Peace through vigilance currently reigns.

CHAPTER 7

Maryanne Watson had not set out to earn a Doctorate degree in Genetic Biology. She just sort of drifted into it. Doing graduate work was easier than working a real job. Mommy and Daddy were happy to pay for her continuing education. They constantly bragged about how well their little girl was doing.

She led an ivory tower existence. By and large academics were courteous, respectful people. Nobody went homeless and crime was practically non-existent. Promotion to Assistant Professor was pretty much automatic once certain criteria had been met.

Maryanne started having problems focusing on her laboratory research. Her mind wandered. Occasionally, she nodded off. She stared out a window for minutes at a time with a blank look on her face. The change in her behavior did not go unnoticed by her co-workers and graduate students.

The head of the Biology Department, Professor Dalton, called Maryanne into his office. Both the quality and the volume of her research had steadily dropped over the past several months. "Are you experiencing any problems in your personal life?" he asked.

"Yes, both my father and my mother died in a horrible collision with a big rig on the New Jersey Turnpike two months ago," Maryanne explained. "I had to identify their bodies at the morgue. There was a closed casket funeral."

Professor Dalton expressed his sympathies and suggested Maryanne see a psychiatrist. The university would pay for weekly visits. Also, she was entitled to take a leave of absence. Maryanne was welcome to confer with Professor Dalton whenever she felt the need to do so.

***

Dr. Maryanne Watson had grown up in the two-story white with brown trim house on the corner of Western and Pine in Elizabeth, New Jersey. This house held a mixed bag of memories for her—some of them warm and fuzzy, but most of them hurtful, buried deep within her subconscious. The real estate agent had already sold the house. Now, it was up to Maryanne to sort through its contents, separating the wheat from the chaff.

All that remained was the attic. Being summer, it was poorly ventilated, hot and dusty, full of boxes, suitcases, and steamer trunks that would soon be headed for the dumpster. A white rectangular metal box caught her eye. It was the Gilbert chemistry set her older brother, Brad, had received for his fourteenth birthday. Not bothering to read the instructions, Brad had dissolved nails, poisoned pill bugs, and caused a small explosion before his father had took it away from him and hid it in the attic. Prior to her brother's experimentation, Maryanne had shown no interest in science. That all changed following the explosion. It was enough for Brad and the rest of the family to know that Brad had screwed up. Maryanne could not rest until she knew the *how* and *why* of it. Thus began Maryanne's career as a scientist and Brad's career as an explosive expert in the United States Army Special Forces.

There was more to Maryanne's initial interest in Biology than that. Biology seemed safer than Chemistry. As far as she knew, Biology did not involve poisoning or explosions. She remembered having questioned at the time why her parents had chosen to buy her brother a Chemistry set rather than a Microbiology set.

Maryanne had liked microbiology ever since she got an "A+" in it in tenth grade. It had led to a career in genetics. Her current research involved using CRISPR to alter DNA. CRISPR had been around for several decades. Any reasonably intelligent high school senior could master it. In fact, there were rudimentary CRISPR sets for sale on the internet for $150.

Sitting cross-legged on a filthy attic floor staring at a rusting Chemistry set made her realize why she was having difficulty concentrating on the job. Brad had never bothered to read the instructions. She, on the other hand, always did things by the book. In the case of CRISPR that involved making the same repetitive motions over and over ad infinitum. Maryanne was **BORED** stiff. At this point she would welcome an explosion to alter the routine. As Albert Einstein said, "The definition of insanity is doing the same thing over and over again and expecting a different result." The scientific method was originally meant to be fluid. Terrified of making a mistake, large educational institutions are crippling genetic innovation.

What to do about it? All business involves risk. The greater the risk, the greater the reward. Maryanne now saw her life's work as creating, manufacturing, and popularizing a genetic biology set. High time to bring new ideas and new blood to CRISPR research.

What to do about it? All business involves risk. The greater the risk, the greater the reward. Maryanne now saw her life's work as creating, manufacturing, and popularizing a genetic biology set. High time to bring new ideas and new blood to CRISPR research.

Dutifully, Maryanne discussed her notion of producing and promoting a CRISPR genetic biology set with the university administrator in charge of biological research. He said the university was not interested in such matters. Dr. Watson would do better by paying closer attention to her research rather than following distractive, unproductive tangents which would ultimately prove unimportant.

Maryanne was not deterred. Over the course of the next few months, she presented her idea to five CEO's of companies which specialized in educational aids. Three turned her down flat. The fourth strung her along.

Something must be wrong, but what could it be? She believed she had perfected her pitch. There must be something else wrong with her presentation. Possibly what was needed was a finished product complete with instructions. She bought a surplus industrial first aid kit online. Its metal box was ideal for what she had in mind. Maryanne spray painted the box bright white inside and out. Then, with an artist's brush and a half pint of scarlet acrylic paint, she wrote in large, bold stylized block letters across the front: **DOCTOR WATSON'S CRISPR GENETIC BIOLOGY KIT**. The most difficult part was writing the instructions and suggested experiments. The experiments had to be both interesting and 100 percent safe.

Maryanne's next presentation was to a middle aged female CEO. It seemed to be going well. To finalize the deal and make certain that the CRISPR kits would be available in stores and online for the Christmas season, she offered to invest $6,500 in the project.

Maryanne was in line for but never obtained tenure at the university. When next year's budget for the university was passed, Maryanne was furloughed. She had half expected it. Doctor Watson's CRISPR Biology sets were now on retail stores' shelves. Time to exit her day job. Time to line up appearances on television and internet talk shows and do everything she could to promote the product.

CHAPTER 8

Benny Evans was a product of the foster care system. In his 17 years, he had been passed around like a migrant worker. Six months here, two years there, with no place he could point to as home. He wasn't even sure Evans was his last name. When in doubt, social workers have been known to make up a name.

For the last two years, Benny had been living with the Andersons and their 14 year old cat, Rufus, in a tract home in Garden Grove, California. Most of the families in the foster care business were in it for the money. Not so the Andersons. Following a successful bout with ovarian cancer, Mrs. Betty Anderson had a hysterectomy. Caring for foster children helped to assuage her maternal instincts.

The Andersons had discussed adopting Benny, but adoption had never progressed beyond talk. Benny knew that children beyond the age of six stood little chance of being adopted. Most couples opted to adopt an infant. Even then, the "cute kids" got placed first. Benny figured his olive skin and broad nose labeled him a mutt. If an animal mutt was not adopted from the pound within a certain period of time, he was put to sleep. But human mutts simply remained a ward of the court until their eighteenth birthday when they were tossed out into the street. A few were emancipated by the court before they reached the age of majority, but they had to have a steady job, a place to live, and a clean arrest record.

***

Benny was by no means a stellar scholar. In fact, he ranked in the bottom third of his class. Last semester, he got a "D" in English and a "C" in Math. He had little interest in academics and even less in sports. Biology was more his speed. Since Day One in Bio Lab when he used a scalpel to slice a flatworm down the middle to the consternation of Ruth, his lab partner, who promptly vomited on the instructor, he found the subject fascinating. Three weeks later, he dismembered a frog, labeling all of the parts correctly which earned both Benny and Ruth an "A" for the course.

Christmas was coming. For most foster families Christmas meant cheap gifts from the dollar store, but the Andersons were different. Last Christmas, they had gifted him a ten speed mountain bike. This Christmas, Benny was asking for Doctor Watson's CRISPR Biology set.

The Andersons did not disappoint Benny. On Christmas morning, he woke up, put on a bathrobe, and went downstairs. There under the decorated six foot blue spruce Christmas tree was a large dazzlingly white metal box with Doctor Watson's CRISPR Biology Set written across the front and a red satin bow on top.

"Thank you, this is the best Christmas ever," exclaimed Benny as they had a family hug. Little did they know that for the rest of the world, this day would live in infamy.

The CRISPR Biology Set fit neatly under Benny's bed. It was as if it had been custom made for Benny Evans. The best part about it was that he could use it at night with the Andersons being none the wiser.

Benny carefully read the instructions and did two experiments before he acquired confidence in using the equipment. He began to design his own experiments, some of which would have been frowned upon by serious scientists.

Benny felt that society regarded him as a nobody, meant to be kicked around under the foster care system until he turned 18 at which time the government could wash their hands of him. He needed to do something momentous soon, something grand which would draw attention to himself. The thing at which he was best was altering DNA. Benny had read about the Japanese man, Mr. Seto who created the three monsters who ravaged parts of Southern California seven years ago. It had taken Mr. Seto years to plan and execute his project. Benny didn't have that long. Benny's best bet was to do something relatively simple with DNA that would grab people's attention.

The simplest thing to do genetically would be to alter RNA which is a single-stranded molecule in many of its biological roles and consists of much shorter chains of nucleotides. Most viruses fit into this category. Benny needed a virus with punch, something that would make the Center for Disease Control stand up and take notice. He thought about resurrecting smallpox. No, that was gruesome. Besides, bringing back smallpox might end up with him sharing a jail cell with Mr. Seto or worse.

But wait. There are two forms of smallpox virus, variola

major and variola minor. Infection with variola major can prove fatal (thirty percent death rate). However, variola minor rarely results in death (less than one percent death rate). Maybe he could transform variola minor into a new and separate virus, variola medium, that would pose an intermediate danger. Surely, that would make his name and earn him fame within the scientific community.

Benny went on the dark web and found an anonymous person who was willing to sell him a sample of variola minor virus. It came with a genome listing approximately 200 genes or gene vestiges, of which slightly under half were identical.

The attributes of some of the genes were known, but most were unknown. Benny bought a dozen white mice on which to test his genetic edits. Gene editing was largely hit or miss. In other words, each separate action had to be tested for effect. It was a long, tedious process. Sometimes he had to make do. For instance, a real, properly funded laboratory would most likely use primates for testing at various points.

Three months of editing and testing resulted in an altered virus which appeared to meet Benny's specifications for a variola medium virus. Due to Benny's limited means, there was a possibility of a ludicrously large margin of error in its rate of contagion.

Benny Evans filled four small vials with his variola medium virus. One would be mailed to the Center for Disease Control (CDC) together with a letter of explanation and the other three would later be placed in liquid nitrogen to preserve them for future experimentation.

Glancing at his wristwatch, Benny saw that he would be late for school if he didn't hurry. He placed the four vials of virus on top of a chest of drawers, grabbed his backpack, and exited out the bedroom door, neglecting to close it completely.

***

8:15 AM and the Andersons were out the front door headed for work. 8:30 AM and Benny was running down the sidewalk to catch the bus to school. Yet another morning that Rufus had to himself to do whatever he chose to do.

Morning sunshine streamed in through the kitchen window. Catnap time. Rufus leaped and landed on the window sill, sprawling along its inclined ledge so as to get the maximum benefit from the sun's rays.

T wo hours later, a pigeon pecking at a window pane woke Rufus up. *Stupid bird!* Catnap definitely over. Time to explore. Nothing new in the bathroom. Nothing new in the hallway. Taking the carpeted steps two at a time, Rufus effotlessly leaped upstairs. *Bedroom door open.* Rufus sauntered on in, tail held high. He spotted the four small vials atop the dresser drawers. *Cat toys!* Rufus jumped on Benny's unmade bed from which he was able to leap to the top of the dresser drawers. He batted the vials one by one onto the floor. *No more fun here.* Rufus went back downstairs for a final catnap before the family came home.

Benny was the first to get home. He no sooner went upstairs to his room than he noticed the vials were missing.

No, not missing, he spotted two on the floor and a quick search on his hands and knees yielded a third under the bed.

A squeaky board on the stairs alerted Benny that Mr. Anderson was home and coming upstairs.

"What are you doing on your knees" asked Mr. Anderson as he stood in the doorway to Benny's bedroom. "Praying? Or are you scrubbing that filthy floor? Why didn't you make up your bed this morning?"

"Sorry, I woke up late for school this morning," explained Benny Evans. "I am looking for something that I dropped on the floor."

"Tell me what you dropped and I will help you look for it," offered Mr. Anderson, entering Benny's bedroom. As he did so, he brushed against the partially open door which freed the missing vial that had become lodged in the small gap between the door and the floor. The heretofore missing virus vial slowly rolled across the bedroom floor. Mr. Anderson's second step crushed the plastic vial, smashing it into smithereens.

Benny was spot on for the lethality rate for variola medium. It fell somewhere between the death rate for variola major and the death rate for variola minor. However, his calculations for the rate of contagion were flawed. Fully seventy percent of the people who came into close contact with someone who had variola medium became infected themselves. Over the course of three weeks after its accidental release, variola medium became a nationwide epidemic. Within three months, it grew into a global pandemic.

Mr. and Mrs. Anderson were among the first to come down with variola medium, but they both recovered rapidly. Benny Evans was sent to a rural Juvenile facility and released on his eighteenth birthday. Due to a legal technicality, he was not prosecuted as an adult. It is rumored that he now works for the CDC. Rufus still takes regular catnaps. Following their recovery, the Andersons bought him a new set of cat toys.

CHAPTER 9

Two months prior to finishing his residency at the Whyte Clinic, Dr. Ostrowski applied for a permanent position with the Center for Disease Control and was hired three weeks later without a face-to-face interview. The CDC wasn't his first choice, but it paid well and held the prospect that after five years of service, his student loans would be forgiven.

He would be working as an infectious disease epidemiologist, confirming the outbreak and presence of disease and advising local public officials of how to deal with it (both domestically and abroad). Needless to say, the job involved a large amount of travel for which he would hopefully be reimbursed.

Dr. Ostrowski's first assignment was in Southern California where he would be organizing the fight against a previously unknown virus resembling smallpox. The mystery virus was so new that it had not yet been given a name. The first few cases originated in a small upscale area of two story tract homes. None of the victims had recently been abroad. It made no sense, new viruses did not normally pop-up out of nowhere.

At noon the next day, Dr. Ostrowski received a phone call from a CDC administrator identifying the virus as having been man made. A vial of the virus had been mailed to the CDC along with a note stating that it had been created by a high school student using a commercially available CRISPR Biology set. For the time being the Center for Disease Control wanted to keep the matter confidential.

The point of origin of the outbreak was determined to be the Anderson's home. Following their recovery, the Andersons were extensively interviewed and the existence of Benny's CRISPR Biology set was made known. Benny was arrested and his Biology set was confiscated as evidence. Two vials of the virus were missing. Benny Evans was either unwilling or unable to account for them.

Dr. Ostrowski directed the unsuccessful search of the Anderson's home for the two missing vials by CDC workers in haz mat suits and respirators. However, Benny's journal in which he recorded his experiments was found on the top shelf of a closet in his bedroom. A week later, the house was tented and fumigated by order of a federal judge.

Covering one wall of the CDC Virulent Virus Task Force's office is a large three county street map with red pins marking individual infections, orange pins indicating multiple cases at the same address, and black pins indicating deaths. It is the primary duty of one CDC worker to keep this chart up to date. Two other workers man the phone lines, interviewing victims, informing those who may have come into contact with someone infected with the virus, and maintaining statistics. Two more workers are in charge of ordering and distributing ventilators, supplies, and related items. A refrigerator big rig truck is parked nearby to handle overflow from the morgue should it become necessary.

An undisclosed source in the federal government leaked

a copy of Benny Evans' journal to the Washington Post parts of which were published. Thus, the new virus came to be popularly known by the name its creator, Benny Evans gave it: variola medium.

Smallpox was declared eradicated by the World Health Organization (WHO) in 1980. However, two samples for research purposes still exist. One is stored in a laboratory in Atlanta, Georgia, the other in Russia. Due to the similarities between variola major and variola medium, interest has been renewed in studying variola major. Unfortunately, a Russian biologist inadvertently exposed a Siberian village to smallpox, a fact which Russia denies. It has spread to Wuhan, China, where the death toll is currently nearing one thousand. Individual cases have been identified in Malaysia and the Philippines.

CRISPR editing has permitted humankind to encroach on roles that were formerly the exclusive preserve of God. The sad part is that overall we haven't been doing that good of a job at it. Given time, perhaps we will learn. Until then, we will have to rely on international institutions such as the World Health Organization and the Center for Disease Control to regulate our behavior.

CHAPTER 10

Dr. Ostrowski had been in charge of the CDC's Variola Medium Task Force for slightly more than a year. During that time he had seen the rate of infection drop from more than 1,000 new cases per day to less than one per week. Social distancing had been discontinued and wearing face masks was no longer mandatory. Supermarket shelves were once again fully stocked, professional sports had staged a remarkable comeback, bars and restaurants had reopened, gymnasiums were building bodies, tattoo parlors were staining skin, and beauty salons were servicing their clientele.

The Variola medium epidemic appeared to have played itself out. Then something unanticipated happened. Orange County General Hospital admitted a twenty-seven year old migrant farm worker exhibiting Variola medium symptoms. However, the test he took for the disease came back negative. The virus had mutated. Over the next few days, pustules appeared over 95 percent of his body. His internal organs began to shutdown. Thirteen days later, he died. The cause of death on the death certificate was listed by the attending physician as "multiple complications from what is suspected to be a novel strain of the Variola medium virus."

The Governor of California went on record calling the new virus "Variola medium 2.0. Its one saving grace was that it died at temperatures of less than 37 degrees. Unfortunately, so did several frail and elderly patients when they were exposed to the cold for an extended period of time.

Would the virus 2.0 mutate again? "Most likely," replied a CDC researcher when asked that question by Dr. Ostrowski. "In its 2.0 mode it appears rather unstable."

Scandinavia, Iceland, Canada, Finland, and other northern climes were spared the brunt of the novel 2.0 pandemic. Tropical and desert areas fared the worst. China, India, and Indonesia instituted one child per family policies as a means of combatting multiple pandemics.

Although the future looked bleak, Dr. Ostrowski forced himself to maintain a positive attitude when being interviewed by the media. His greatest fear was that something he said would spark disorder and panic. Civilization is a thin veneer. Scratch the surface and you may well expose the animal that is man.

Given the destruction and social unrest generated by multiple pandemics, governments, institutions, and the ties that bind were being severely tested. In some cases they completely crumbled. Anarchy ensued. The world economy was not likely to recover anytime soon.

Six months into the variola 2.0 virus J.C. Penney filed Chapter 11 bankruptcy. A host of other retail businesses followed suit. The federal government bailed out domestic auto makers, ostensibly to keep them from laying off their employees.

As if variola 2.0 had not caused enough problems, the large quantity of antibodies produced by five year old and younger victims' systems to combat variola 2.0 were producing symptoms of Kawasaki disease. Due to the danger posed to the heart, these children required hospitalization for extended periods of time.

With multiple pandemics striking simultaneously resources were being stretched thin. Disposable hospital gowns were being sold for seven dollars each and disinfectant was rationed by retailers as to how much a customer would be allowed to buy at one time.

Twenty-five percent of the U.S. workforce were unemployed due to social distancing and shelter in place directives. Not since the Great Depression had so many people been unemployed. Of those still employed, a large percentage were working from home via the internet.

The travel and tourist industries were devastated. Those ocean liners who were not at sea when variola 2.0 struck stayed in port. Those at sea had a difficult time finding a port that would permit them to dock. Airliners operated at 30 percent capacity. Many routes simply weren't being serviced.

With less traffic on the ground, in the air, and on the sea, oil prices plummeted. A worldwide glut of petroleum products sent the price of a barrel of oil into the negative range for the first time in anyone's memory. Environmental activists deemed it the beginning of the end for fossil fuels.

CHAPTER 11

Charity Smythe was a scion of scions dating from when her namesake ancestor stepped onto Plymouth Rock after she disembarked from the Mayflower. Charity's mother served as the President General of the Daughters of the American Revolution, a role which Charity intended to someday inherit.

The debutante ball in which she would be presented to society and Charity's eighteenth birthday happened to coincide. Not wanting to be short of time for preparing for the debutante ball, she tore into a pile of birthday gifts without paying attention to who gave them to her. Most were jewelry (always a safe gift for a young lady of status) or perfume. One exceptionally large gift intrigued her. It was a dazzlingly white metal box with **Doctor Watson's CRISPR Biology Set** emblazoned across the front.

Who would give her such an inappropriate gift? In four years of attending a private prep school for girls she had not taken a single science course. She rummaged through labels, cards, and crumpled wrapping paper in vain, searching for a clue as to the gauche goof who gave it to her.

The following afternoon, Charity placed the Biology set in the rear of her enormous walk-in closet, there, presumably, to await transport to the county dump, along with six pairs of outdated shoes, three torn dresses, a half pint of incredibly cheap perfume in a blue cut glass bottle, and whatever else she chose to discard.

Two months later, Charity was showing some new outfits she had bought on a recent shopping spree at the Mall of America with her mother to her best friend, Cynthia McDonald (yes, **that** McDonald), when Cynthia spotted the Dr. Watson's CRISPR Biology kit lying on the floor in the rear of Charity's walk-in closet.

"I wasn't sure of what to give you for your birthday," Cynthia confessed. "You already have everything a girl could possibly wish for. That is when I thought of getting you a CRISPR kit. I got mine six months ago on the advice of my Biology teacher, Mr. Santee. He's so cute, he drives an Aston Martin Valkyrie, and he's unmarried. Mr. Santee says that CRISPR is already making revolutionary changes in the human race. And we can be part of it. It's not easy, but I intend to master it. But look," Cynthia remarked as she dragged the Biology set into the middle of Charity's bedroom, "there isn't a smudge or a scratch on it. It is as if it hadn't been opened."

"That is because it is one of my most prized possessions," Charity prevaricated. "I keep it spotless. I had the upstairs maid clean it yesterday," Charity intentionally lied with malice aforethought towards all those who earn their living by the sweat of their brows. "Those filthy little buggy creatures dirty everything. It's a wonder anyone wants to become a biologist."

"I want to be a biologist. Specifically, I intend to become a geneticist," Cynthia declared. "CRISPR will enable us to increase our intelligence, eliminate disease, and achieve immortality. Improved harvests of genetically modified crops will make hunger a thing of the past. Our descendants will be Masters of the Universe. It all starts here," Cynthia exclaimed while drumming her fingers on **Doctor Watson's CRISPR Biology Set**.

Charity had never known her friend to lie. Clearly, Cynthia intended to spark a new interest in science. Perhaps such a trend had been a long time coming. Fads regularly come and go. In order to remain fashionable trend setters are among the first in and the first to move on to the next trend. Charity and her entourage would gain everything worth gaining from this new social media topic, at least until it peaked.

"Um...m...m...m...m...Masters of the Universe," chortled Charity to no one in particular shortly after Cynthia had left. The CRISPR Biology set remained in the center of the bedroom. Rather than drag it back into the closet, Charity decided she would open it. After all, if this kit contained the power to make someone the Master of the Universe, it was definitely worth a look-see.

The first thing Charity noticed as she opened The CRISPR Biology set was a thick, heavy Instruction Manual with Suggested Experiments. She spent several minutes browsing through it, rapidly flipping the pages, and occasionally pausing to glance at an illustration. With that over, she tossed the instruction book/manual into a wastebasket. **Doctor Watson's CRISPR Biology Set** was overweight in her opinion. This Dr. Watson fellow needed to get real. Every ounce of deadweight she could shed from it would make it that much easier to move around. Besides, only dummies rely on instructions. The best and the brightest figure things out for themselves.

Not really understanding what she was doing, Charity began by mixing vials together, much as one would do with a chemistry set. To her surprise nothing monumental happened, so she grew bored with it and hauled it back to her closet.

The next day, Charity got together with some of her friends and they were all aglow, telling tales of the successes they were having with their CRISPR biology sets. Not to be outdone, Charity made up a story of how well she was doing with CRISPR. It wasn't the first time she made up a story, nor would it be the last. Knowing Charity as they did everyone refrained from calling her a liar. Charity was known for getting even with those who irritated her. No doubt that is how she came to be the leader of her clique.

In order to be recognized as an authentic part of the CRISPR crowd one had to learn the proper terminology. Thus, when Charity began her first experience with CRISPR by mixing vials of virus together, she was looking to perform an antigenic shift, at least that is how she described it once she got the lingo down pat. Much of the clique's fascination with CRISPR stemmed from the fact that it enabled them to speak over other people's heads. They had the appearance backed up by the lingo that they knew what they were doing. By their values image was everything. Remember, these are girls who dress to impress. Their initial incursion into the scientific community was no doubt spurred by a similar motive, which in no way is meant to demean or discourage them from their activities. It is simply meant as a partial explanation of how things later went wrong.

Cynthia told Charity and the rest of the clique that she had success doing an antigenic shift with a Corona virus.

"But there is no Corona virus in the CRISPR kit," asserted Diana, the newest member of the group.

"Of course not, you ninny, I had to get Corona virus on my own," retorted Cynthia. "I'll tell you what. I've got more Corona virus than I will ever use. I'll bring each of you a vial of it when we get together on Saturday."

"There are a large range of Corona viruses," asserted Diana. "It's a rather large group. Some come from dogs, some from humans, some from cats, and others from who knows where. I mean, I will be grateful for anything I get, but it would help to know where the virus came from."

"Well, smarty, if you must know, I bought it from this spooky fellow I met on the internet. He wouldn't tell me where he lives, but the extension on his email address makes me think he lives in China. It's either that or he is routing his messages through a series of bots or whatnot. He had me pay him in crypytocurrency, as if we were dealing illegal drugs," explained Cynthia. "Mr. Spooky sent me twenty-three vials of the stuff. He said it came from bats."

"Ugh, bats are creepy," exclaimed Charity. "They bite the back of your neck, suck out all your blood, and turn you into one of Dracula's minions. Definitely not for me."

"Oh, God, give me strength. It's not like you will be coming into contact with bats or any other animal for that matter," Cynthia countered, throwing up her hands while bowing her head to add emphasis to what she was saying. "CRISPR Biologists work in a sanitized, temperature controlled environment. It is the last place in the world where something could sneak up on you and bite you on the neck."

With that the gathering began breaking up. It was clear that Cynthia was challenging Charity for leadership of the clique and nobody wanted to stick around to witness the outcome. Besides, the tension was more drama than reality; a clash of egos not likely to have any lasting effect. Charity and Cynthia had been best friends for as long as anyone could remember. Despite occasional flare-ups, that was not likely to change. This type of social interaction could be expected from upper crust young ladies with far too much free time on their hands.

***

Mr. Spooky had not been entirely forthcoming with Cynthia. What he failed to disclose was that the bat Corona virus he sold her came with SARs receptor, a potentially pathological combination, which explains why he wanted to dispose of it in a manner that left no possibility of it being traced back to him.

In an effort to accelerate scientific processing on developing next year's influenza vaccine (an annual project with a rigid deadline that is both outsourced and funded by American Big Pharma), biohazard security at a Wuhan University laboratory where Mr. Spooky was employed as a laboratory technician had relaxed enforcement, with the result that a virulent Corona virus Mr. Spooky had been genetically modifying was now infecting the locals, spreading rapidly, and threatening to become an epidemic. If the proper measures to contain the Corona virus were not put into place soon, it could multiply into a pandemic with devastating consequences for humanity, the social order, and the global economy. No doubt heads would roll. Mr. Spooky was doing everything he could to obfuscate his role in the debacle and make certain that his head would not be among them. The communist Government of the People's Republic of China would be merciless with anybody deemed responsible for having harmed the social order. In this case the damage was massive and ongoing.

***

It was evident from the manner in which the clique discussed CRISPR that they had little idea of how dangerous it could be in the hands of amateurs. However, a note of caution did surface at their next meeting only to be mercilessly quashed by Cynthia as she doled out the contaminated vials of Corona virus.

"Are you completely certain that this virus is safe?" asked Diana as Cynthia handed her a vial.

"Absolutely. It came by mail from halfway around the world. Do you think that our government is so stupid that they would let these vials into the United States without testing them to see if they posed a threat? Maybe before 9/11, but definitely not now. No doubt Homeland Security x-rayed, fluoroscoped, and had sniffer dogs examine the package before they turned it over to the Postal Service to deliver to my door," pontificated Cynthia, scowling at Diana for having questioned authority once too often.

Following suit, the rest of the girls in the clique shot Diana dirty looks. How dare the new girl question the character of a founding member of the clique?

***

In addition to fighting the variola virus, the CDC Virulent Virus Task Force is responsible for monitoring and limiting the spread of related contagious diseases such as influenza. Tracing influenza's course through the population occasionally reveals hot spots which require special attention. However, one hot spot located in the heart of a Southern California upper class community proved particularly difficult to analyze and control. A never-before-seen strain of influenza struck multiple homes at once and could not be traced back to a single source.

Due to the mysterious influenza virus' unique nature and the social clout of its victims, Dr. Ostrowski was directed by his superiors at the Center for Disease Control to personally take charge of a high priority investigation into the origin of the outbreak.

Due to the mysterious influenza virus' unique nature and the social clout of its victims, Dr. Ostrowski was directed by his superiors at the Center for Disease Control to personally take charge of a high priority investigation into the origin of the outbreak.

Because the influenza virus outbreak was concentrated in a relatively small area, Dr. Ostrowski decided to go door to door, interviewing as many people as possible. It was grueling work for a physician not accustomed to pounding the pavement, but such are the rigors of collecting evidence in an investigation.

'Have you recently returned from a trip abroad?' 'Is anyone in your family running a fever or is there anyone who has difficulty breathing?' 'Have you recently been around someone who was coughing either at home or at work?' Dr. Ostrowski repeated these questions and others to each person he interviewed in the attempt to get a handle on the Corona virus.

Although polite, the residents were not forthcoming. Dr. Ostrowski began each interview by identifying himself, displaying his credentials, and stating the official nature and purpose of his visit. By the time he had gone to twenty-five houses, he began to think that people were suspicious of him. Also, he had the impression that someone was phoning their neighbors, warning them that a government agent who might possibly quarantine their community was going door-to-door.

Because he was getting nowhere fast, Dr. Ostrowski decided to change his approach. He quit scaring people with the possibility of mandatory quarantine and added that all answers would be kept in strict confidence. Dr. Ostrowski stressed that he was concerned with the community's welfare; he was in no way associated with law enforcement. The people being interviewed became less suspicious. A few offered him something to drink. One even invited him inside to conduct the interview. However, early in the afternoon, it all came to an end when Owen failed to notice a female Chihuahua nursing her puppies in a cardboard box on a porch. As he was ringing the doorbell, he had his back to her. The small mother dog bit him hard through his sock twice on his left ankle, breaking the skin both times. Evidently, no one was home because nobody answered the door. Also, there were a number of newspapers strewn around the front lawn and several fliers hanging from the front doorknob. So ended the first day's investigation.

Bandaged but wiser, on the second day, Dr. Ostrowski gave up his expensive brown wing tips for a pair of comfortable hiking boots. He had not gone two blocks when he hit pay dirt.

When he knocked on the front door, a teenage girl came to the door. Since both of her parents were working and would not be home until after dark, he showed her his credentials and asked her if she wouldn't mind answering a few questions, the answers to which would be used in a government health survey to combat a contagious virus that was threatening the community. He had no more jotted down her name and address when he looked through the screen door and saw a familiar item propped against one wall in the living room.

"Excuse me, Miss, but I couldn't help noticing the large white metal chest sitting on the floor inside the door," observed Dr. Ostrowski. "Isn't that a CRISPR Biology set?"

"Why, yes it is," replied the teenaged girl, glancing back at the item in question. "I belong to a club that is currently focusing on genetics. I'm applying to a number of colleges. Vassar is my first choice. They have a strong program in Biology."

"I have some experience with CRISPR myself, however, my experience occurred in a state-of-the-art laboratory under supervision. It was a rather time-consuming, complicated process. Of course, that was years ago. I see Dr. Watson has simplified CRISPR to the point where it can be used at home by a high school Biology student," deduced Dr. Ostrowski. "Would you mind if I took a look at what is inside of it?"

"My parents gave me strict orders not to let anyone in the house until they get home," blurted out the Vassar applicant.

"And well they should," Dr. Ostrowski replied with emphasis. "It seems we share a common interest. You could let me open it here on the porch."

"It's rather heavy," she hedged.

"That should pose no difficulty for a young, athletic girl like yourself. You do know that a letter of appreciation from the Center for Disease Control would help you get admitted to Vassar?," suggested Dr. Ostrowski. "I could write it myself and have the Director of CDC sign it."

"You'd do that for me? You hardly know me," she said as she lugged the CRISPR Biology set from the living room onto the front porch.

"From the questionnaire I know your name is Diana Dumont. I appreciate that you are helping me find the source of a terrible virus that is afflicting this community," Dr. Ostrowski stated as he opened the brass clasps that kept the CRISPR set closed. There among the test tubes, petri dishes, pipettes, tubing, and clear translucent vials was a single yellow opaque vial that wasnâ €™t part of the set. Owen had a hunch that he was about to solve the mystery surrounding the origin of this outbreak.

"May I borrow this?," Dr. Owen Ostrowski asked as he held up the suspicious yellow vial in his right hand.

"Sure you can," replied Diana who was all smiles. *She was going to Vassar!*

"By the way, I will be returning tonight to talk to your parents and get their answers to the questionnaire," commented Dr. Ostrowski as he pocketed the yellow vial, turned around, and stepped off the Dumont household's front porch, intent on returning to the Virulent Virus Task Force's office posthaste in order to analyze the contents of the yellow, opaque vial.

* * *

"Good evening, Mr. Dumont. My name is Dr. Ostrowski and I am with the Center for Disease Control. There has been a Corona virus flareup in your neighborhood and I am trying to get to the bottom of it. I talked to your daughter earlier in the day and now I have come back to interview you and your wife. It will only take a few minutes of your time."

"Diana already told me what happened," asserted Mr. Dumont, blocking the doorway with his ample body to prevent the doctor from barging his way in. "My attorney says that taking something from a minor child under false pretenses is a prosecutable offense. Nor would a criminal court permit you to introduce that Godforsaken vial. Shame on you, getting her hopes up for being admitted to Vassar."

"I am a CDC doctor interviewing people in order to track and eliminate a deadly virus. In no way am I connected with law enforcement," Dr. Ostrowski reiterated as he took an envelope from his breast pocket. "The CDC is concerned with public health, not fixing blame. Diana is a hero. She saved countless lives and millions of dollars by helping to identify the source of the Corona virus that is infecting your community and spreading like wildfire." Handing Mr. Dumont an envelope, Dr. Ostrowski waited while Diana's protectful father opened it and read:

LETTER OF APPRECIATION

The Center for Disease Control appreciates the assistance and continuing cooperation of Ms. Diana Dumont without whose help in identifying the source of an outbreak of toxic Corona virus in her community, countless lives and millions of dollars would have been lost.

Diana Dumont is a true American hero, proof positive that many young people are on the right track to build a brighter, better future, free of disease in which humankind can prosper.

Our field operative tells me that Diana aspires to be admitted to Vassar where she wants to major in Biology. I, speaking for the entire CDC, wish her success.

The world owes Ms. Diana Dumont its gratitude,

Myrtle H. Redfern, Director, Centers for Disease Control

"That Letter of Appreciation was faxed to me less than an hour before I came here. I know of no other young person who has received a similar commendation," summed up Dr. Ostrowski.

"Alright, I got you wrong. You are who you say you are and from what I have seen you are leveling with us," confessed Mr. Dumont. "It just didn't seem likely that a doctor would go door to door."

"I don't particularly enjoy pounding the pavement, but until I talked with Diana, it was necessary to wear out some shoe leather in an attempt to learn how the Corona virus outbreak got started. The next step is to contain it before it gets beyond control. For that I need your family's continuing cooperation," Dr. Ostrowski requested.

"Please come in," backtracked Mr. Dumont, standing aside and throwing the front door fully open. "Have a seat and tell me how we can help you fight this dreaded virus."

"First, I need for all three of you and anyone you employ as a housekeeper, maintenance man, or gardener to be tested for the Corona virus at CDC expense. Second, I need the names of anyone whom each of you has come in contact with during the past two weeks. I also need the names and phone numbers of everyone in the club that Diana joined. Place an asterisk beside those who own a CRISPR kit; two asterisks for people who have one or more of the yellow vials; three asterisks for the club's leader. Also, jot down anything else that might be relevant to this case," directed Dr. Ostrowski.

"I didn't think that the Biology set would cause trouble when I bought it for Diana. Now, I wish I had never seen it. I am going to throw it in a dumpster," Mr. Dumont stated.

"Don't do that," cautioned Dr. Ostrowski. "The CRISPR Biology set is safe as long as the instruction booklet is followed. There are some bad actors on social media who are encouraging young people to do things they shouldn't be doing. Since Diana did not break the seal on the yellow vial, I doubt she had any part in the Corona virus outbreak. Diana is going to be a top-notch biologist. Maybe someday she will win a Nobel Prize. In the meantime, you need to give her the right kind of encouragement and supervision."

The next morning, one of Dr. Ostrowski's assistants picked up the contact list of names from the Dumont family. She divided the list into four more or less equal parts, each of which was given to a Center for Disease Control field worker whose job it was to trace the path of the Corona virus, inhibiting the progress of the virus wherever possible.

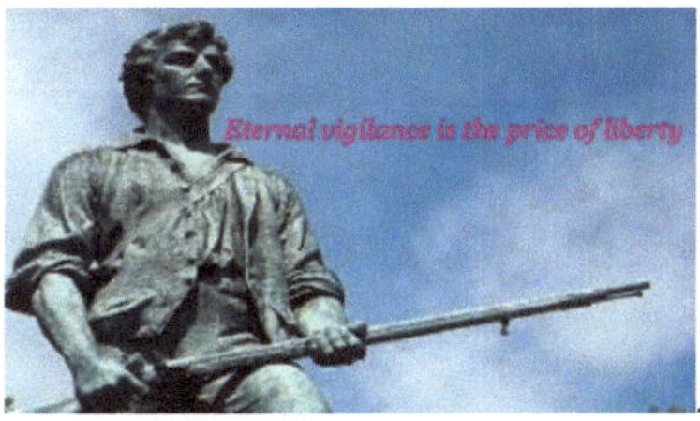

As for Dr. Ostrowski, he was busy writing a report about the outbreaks in his area, stressing the foreign GMO origin of the Corona with SAR's receptor virus which was being introduced into cities across the United States via false and/or misleading videos on social media. He boldly concluded that the current wave of epidemics and pandemics which were negatively affecting global health and commerce were manmade rather than a result of the forces of nature. The Free World is under attack by totalitarian forces eeking to undermine democracy through malevolent misinformation transmitted by social media as well as CRISPR-associated biological warfare directed at civilian populations. This two prong ongoing sneak attack had already done more damage and claimed more lives than Pearl Harbor and 9/11 combined, but neither our leaders nor the American public recognizes it for what it is. Once again, we are reminded that eternal vigilance is the price of liberty.

CHAPTER 12

Although still in charge of the Virulent Virus Task Force, Dr. Ostrowski was temporarily recalled to CDC headquarters in Atlanta, Georgia, presumably to discuss his report in greater detail. When he was hired the previous year, he had been under the mistaken impression that his job would be to treat people infected with contagious disease. Actually, his job turned out to be more of an advisory and investigative nature. Travel was not his forte. From what little experience he had acquired, he was of the opinion that if you had seen one major U.S. metropolis, you had pretty much seen them all.

However, Atlanta was different in one respect. After social distancing, wearing face masks, closing businesses, and taking all of the CDC recommended precautions when a virulent virus was first detected in Georgia three months ago, Georgia's Governor got antsy and eliminated restrictions despite CDC advice to the contrary. Now, Georgia was paying the price in terms of deaths that could have been prevented had the proper measures been kept in place. Dr. Ostrowski was concerned about traveling to Atlanta in the midst of a resurgent pandemic for something which could (and as Owen saw it should) have been done via a conference call on Skype.

A line from Alfred Lord Tennyson's poem, The Charge of the Light Brigade, kept popping up in the restless doctor's mind as he tried to fall asleep in the antebellum downtown Atlanta hotel room the CDC had booked for him: "Ours not to reason why, ours but to do and die." Sleep eluded him for hours. Finally, a scene from Gone with the Wind in which Atlanta burned down to the ground brought him much needed REM sleep. Waking blurry-eyed at 6:30 AM in the morning when the alarm clock on the nightstand next to his bed began to beep, he could not help but think, 'If General Sherman had done a better job of torching downtown Atlanta, I probably wouldn't be needlessly risking my life staying in this Godforsaken disease-ridden urban backwater for the next three days.'

Several hours later, while still wearing his monogramed white terrycloth bathrobe and slippers, Dr. Ostrowski heard a knock at the door. Thinking it was room service from which he had ordered lunch shortly before, he quickly opened the door. He was surprised to see a uniformed courier from a messenger service who gave him a note requesting his presence at a CDC executive board meeting at 10:30 AM the next day.

***

When an executive secretary ushered Dr. Ostrowski into the CDC Board Room, it was already 10:45 AM. The Members of the Board were seated on one side of a long polished table in leather swivel chairs with the Chairman of the Board smack dab in the middle presiding over proceedings while sitting comfortably in an overstuffed cushy Corinthian leather throne. Dr. Ostrowski took a seat in the middle of the other side of the table in a hardwood straight back library chair which from the initials carved into two of its legs and the rock hard pink bubble gum parked beneath the chair seemed out of place in the sterile, immaculate board room.

After opening the meeting with a wooden gavel, the Chairman coldly stared across the table at Dr. Ostrowski and remarked, "you are late."

"My apologies to the Board. There was a horrible three car accident with injuries that happened in front of me three blocks from here. I stopped to help until several ambulances and a fire truck arrived. After all, my primary duty as a physician is to assist the public. Perhaps you heard the sirens?," Dr. Ostrowski explained.

"Dr. Ostrowski's report and recommendations are the main item on today's agenda," commented the Chairman. "Does everyone have a copy?," he asked. Since no one responded, he continued, "As you all probably know, Dr. Ostrowski heads the Virulent Virus Task Force which has traced an outbreak of the Corona virus with SAR's receptor in Southern California back to its malicious Chinese origin. I say malicious because Dr. Ostrowski has confiscated 23 vials of the virus after it entered the United States through international mail and was about to be distributed to various localities via social media. I have alerted Homeland Security. The matter is now in their hands. The CDC, our nation, and the entire Free World owe Dr. Ostrowski a debt of gratitude. Following a three month lockdown, the United States is experiencing a tremendous surge in the number of new Corona virus cases with outbreaks simultaneously occurring in multiple states. Dr. Ostrowski believes we are under biological attack. After careful study of the evidence and an extensive examination of the Task Force's documentation, CDC Director, Myrtle Redfern, and I have reached a similar conclusion. Dear God please help us! I am confident that our faith will see us through."

Dr. Ostrowski was both surprised and elated at the praise the Chairman heaped on him and his report.

That is, until Gerhart Nunec, the Vice-President for Public Relations, spoke up: "Dr. Ostrowski, you do realize that there are other considerations which must be taken into account when composing a document for public consumption other than statement of facts and documentation. It is imperative that the CDC is seen as taking an apolitical stance towards every issue. We are funded by Congress. Both the legislative and the executive branches of the federal government are currently controlled by a party which for whatever reason chooses to ignore biological and cyber attacks against our nation and pooh-poohs climate change. If we publish this report as is with its questionable allegations and conclusions, we will be committing economic suicide. Any CDC appropriations would be blocked by the Senate. Nary a zinc penny would be forthcoming. We don't want to suffer the same fate as the World Health Organization whose funding was completely cut off by our President. This report should be made public, but not without extensive revisions. Our mission must continue to be disease control and prevention. Public health is our overriding concern.

"Health is the overriding concern of all Americans, but public health is not an absolute. It is influenced by many factors, some of which are civil unrest, poverty, and the environment," countered Dr. Ostrowski. My report provides documented proof that foreign forces are employing biological weaponry in an ongoing multi-pronged sneak attack against the United States. In good conscience and as patriots, we cannot sit back on our haunches and permit this to happen. Japanese forces killed 2,300 Americans in the December 7, 1941 attack on Pearl Harbor that prodded Congress to declare war on Japan. Contrast that statistic with the fact that 125,000 Americans have died as a result of the ongoing biological attack. Moreover, it's getting worse. In 41 of 50 states the daily number of people infected by the Corona virus is on the rise."

"If a firebug is setting fires, get rid of the firebug and you will be rid of the fires. In my experience, the simplest, common sense approach is the path to follow," Dr. Ostrowski counseled by way of example.

"Excuse me," interrupted Stanley Morgan, Financial Executive Officer for the CDC, seated on the right next to the Chairman. "On page 87 of your report, you single out 'Mr. Smokey' (I take it that is his online name) as the source of the manmade virus. Since your biological attack argument is based solely on the actions of this nefarious individual, I would like to know a lot more about him. What is his real name? Is he a Chinese Communist agent? Where is he based? The more you can tell us about him, the better."

"He's a mystery man," proffered Dr. Ostrowski after taking a drink of ice water from a glass tumbler, "which is what one would expect from someone taking part in covert operations. He's channeling his emails through a number of bots in an attempt to obfuscate his identity. It took a lot of effort by my staff to track him down to Wuhan University in China. Through advertisements and endorsements on social media he is labeling virulent virus as being harmless and selling it to unsuspecting young people who utilize it in CRISPR biology experiments. The return address on the packages he sends to buyers in the United States is an empty lot in Shanghai, China. I have no clue as to the size of this covert operation, but judging from the recent spike in U.S. infections, it's scaling up."

"Are you saying that the Corona virus was originally

developed by Chinese scientists intent on creating an effective biological weapon that would disrupt western democracies?," Mr. Morgan queried.

"Definitely not," Dr. Ostrowski answered. "I believe that Wuhan University was doing research funded by the National Institutes of Health focused on developing a vaccine for the upcoming flu season. When NIH unexpectedly turned off the money tap for the project, security procedures at the lab lapsed, resulting in a Corona virus leak that in time infected much of Wuhan Province. Later, a Chinese official recognized that Corona virus could be weaponized. Duping American high school students via social media into distributing the virus simultaneously to a number of locations throughout the United States was part of a covert operation headed by Mr. Smokey."

Following a moment of silence, the Chairman intervened, "If no one objects, I am terminating further discussion of the report. The Executive Board has been presented with two options on how we should proceed. The first option is to publish the complete report. A possible side effect is that it would anger the current Administration to the point where they might attempt to cut off our funds. The second option would be to either ignore or drastically dilute the report, an option which I believe the Director would abhor. I propose a third option. It is clear that given the current political bias, publishing the report would be tantamount to shooting ourselves in the foot. However, not publishing it would be inviting further outbreaks of the pandemic. What we need is a way to publish the report without incurring risk. I propose that we vote to publish, but only the parts that are politically correct. The rest needs to be redacted. I'm willing to bet that there will be a public outcry for the

CDC to release the complete report as originally written."

"The Board will now vote by show of hands on whether to adopt, subject to the Director's approval, options one two, or three. All in favor of option one raise your hand." A short wait while the Chairman looked around before uttering, "all in favor of option two raise your hand." Another short wait followed by "all in favor of option three raise your hand. The Board's vote is unanimous. The Board has chosen to proceed with option number three."

"May I speak?," exclaimed Dr. Ostrowski. "I apologize to the Board for not following correct parliamentary procedure, but they didn't teach that to us in medical school. There is one item that wasn't in the report that I think deserves the Board's attention. Dr. Watson's CRISPR Biology set is being marketed as a toy in the same manner that Gilbert Chemistry sets were sold in an earlier era. If used as the manufacturer intended, it poses no danger. However, I have first hand knowledge of a group of high school students who are using it to edit viruses, some of which may cause disease in humans. I think we need to lobby Congress to place a warning on the front of the box it comes in, e.g., WARNING: This is not a toy. For use only with adult supervision. My first thought was that it should be banned. However, we don't want to discourage students from studying genetics. I believe it should be marketed to schools as an aid for Biology teachers."

"The CDC should avoid becoming embroiled in partisan politics," Mr. Morgan reminded the Executive Board. "I would much prefer that we voice our concerns to the manufacturer and seek voluntary compliance."

Three other board members spoke in favor of voluntary

compliance. The consensus appeared to be that political bias and legislated compliance should be avoided whenever possible. A vote by the Executive Board confirmed it. This time Dr. Ostrowski did not voice an objection.

"If there is any new business, now is the time to bring it to the Board's attention," the Chairman ordered. [short pause] "No new business? Meeting adjourned." [gavel closes meeting] "Mr. Nunec and Dr. Ostrowski, I would like to see you both in my office in 10 minutes."

***

Fifteen minutes later, Vice-President for Public Relations, Gerhart Nunec and the Chief of the Virulent Virus Task Force, Dr. Owen Ostrowski sat in bucket chairs in front of the Chairman's desk, who was about to address them: "I want you two to collaborate on editing a politically correct redacted version of the report. Your team has one week to prepare it and print 250 copies. Also, print 400 copies of the original report which I will store in my office until such time as the Director tells me to release them to the public. This entails Dr. Ostrowski extending his tour of our Atlanta facility for one week, after which he will resume his duties as Chief of the Virulent Virus Task Force. Any questions?"

"Mr. Nunec can edit the report without my interference. I would prefer to return to the field as soon as possible," declared Dr. Ostrowski.

"And I would prefer to spend next week as an inner city free clinic philanthropist-physician binging on *Noblesse oblige*," quipped the Executive Board Chairman, "but neither of us are likely to realize our preferences any time soon. As my sainted mother used to say, "you might as well wish in one hand and shit in the other."

Owen Ostrowski, feeling depressed and defeated, hailed a taxi that took him 3.7 miles to the downtown Atlanta hotel where he was staying. Exiting the cab, he paid the driver the exact amount shown on the meter.

"The customary tip in the South is 15%," advised the scowling taxi driver.

"You want a tip?," responded Dr. Ostrowski.

"Next time you pick up a fare in the midst of a pandemic, wear a mask. That's a tip that just might save your life."

The paper note taped to the hotel elevator read "Out of Order. After shuffling dejectedly over to the stairway on his left, Owen bounded up the stairs, taking them two at a time, until he reached the right floor. He unlocked the door to his room and flung it open. A maid had emptied the metal trash receptacle that stood beside his nightstand and had inadvertently left it in the middle of the floor between the door and the bed. Owen ran at it and placekicked it over the bed. Next, he kicked off his shoes and fell face down on the bed. Three hours later he awoke feeling fully refreshed. Life could be worse, he told himself, but he could not imagine how.

Bright and early the next day, Dr. Ostrowski met with the Vice-President for Public Relations in Mr. Nunec's spacious office to iron out their disagreement about which parts of the report could be published without risking further funding. At noon, when they broke for lunch, it was already clear that neither of them intended to budge.

When they returned from lunch they tried something new, trading an issue for an issue of equal value. In that way, Dr. Ostrowski was able to publish that the Corona virus was manmade in exchange for blacking out all mention of a cyber sneak attack. However, their progress was negated by a phone call from Owen's mother-in-law in which she disclosed that Owen's wife had tested positive for the Corona virus four days before and was admitted to Little Company of Mary Hospital in Torrance, CA, where she appeared to be recovering nicely.

***

"My wife came down with the Corona virus four days ago. She has been admitted to a hospital in Torrance, California," began Dr. Ostrowski. "I need to get there as soon as possible. Nunec can carry on with editing the report."

"If Nunec is left alone with it, the title page will be the only thing that isn't redacted," countered the Chairman of the Executive Board. Besides, hospitals aren't allowing novel Corona virus patients to see visitors, including spouses."

"But they aren't excluding doctors. I'm a physician first, an epidemiologist second," Dr. Ostrowski retorted.

"Alright, take some time off," relented the Chairman. "But please keep it to the bare minimum needed. There is a pandemic going on. It may sound trite, however, we really do need every trained healthcare worker we can get."

"I won't need more than a couple of days," promised Dr. Ostrowski. "Just enough to satisfy her that I care. I'll be back before most people realize I went."

CHAPTER 13

"I've seen mosquitos as large as hummingbirds and spiders as big as your hand, but a 15 foot tall praying mantis that dines on humans, not only that but a swarm of them descending on Anaheim, California, now that's a tall tale you've been telling," proclaimed Kevin, the barkeep at Surly Sam's Saloon.

"It's all true. I would swear it on a Bible, except that there isn't any to be found at Surly Sam's. The closest thing this place has to a Bible is a nine year old beer-stained girly mag," Lynda Loomis remarked as she leaned over her barstool and picked up a magazine perched tent-like atop a brass railing. Lynda spent her days as a genetic researcher at the Whyte Clinic and her nights sucking suds at Surly Sam's Saloon along with a half dozen other regulars. She prided herself on being a social drinker rather than an alcoholic.

"When Walt Disney and his brother Roy were searching for Southern California acreage on which to build Disneyland back in 1954, Roy approached my uncle, Kenneth Dungan, with a low-ball offer to purchase a portion of his orange groves. Kenneth was insulted by such a miserly bid. Shortly afterwards, a swarm of gigantic praying mantises descended on Anaheim decimating the orange crop. To make ends meet, Kenneth chopped down the orange trees and sold them for firewood that winter at $25 a cord," declared Lynda in a voice loud enough to be heard in the furthest corners of the bar.

"That Fall, Kenneth decided to retire from farming. He sold the Disney Corporation his groves for slightly more than their original offer and made them pay cash. He traveled to Thailand, married a princess, bought a 30 foot teak sailboat, and set course for Tasmania. No one ever heard from him again. Some say a Tasmanian tiger ate him. His first wife, Ruby, claims he caught a nasty sexually transmitted disease from the Siamese princess for which medical science has no cure. Nor have they developed a vaccine" Lynda related. "Now, no port in the world will permit him to dock. If you ask me, he should have stayed married to Ruby, bought himself an assault rifle, and turned them 15 foot tall insects into high protein burgers."

"Damn straight," agreed Dirtbag Dan, the weatherbeaten man in a faux leather jacket sitting to the right of her at the bar. "When life gives you lemons, make lemonade."

"She was talking oranges. She didn't say anything about lemons," corrected Easy Earl from a nearby table where he was drawing caricatures of several inebriated patrons on a napkin.

"It doesn't matter what variety of citrus Lynda was babbling about," Kevin proclaimed. "What matters is that the more sotted she becomes, the more she prevaricates, and the less likely she is to pay her bar tab."

"Speak English," demanded Dirtbag Dan. "Any word with more than ten letters isn't fit to be spoken."

"I said Lynda lies. The more she drinks, the more she lies. We all know that. She has been coming here nightly for years and we know next to nothing about her.

Really, Lynda, do you think anybody believes that crap about how you work at a genetic research lab?," Kevin asked with a sneer while making a rude gesture with his middle finger. "What moron would permit a stumble bum like you to work with fragile lab equipment. You shouldn't be ashamed of scrubbing floors or whatever it is you do to make a living."

"You lowlife bastard. I already had a Masters degree in Biology when you were sniffing little girls' panties in first grade," Lynda shouted as she slid off the barstool and struggled to standup straight. "You have insulted me for the last time," Lynda swore, with the sound of hysterical laughter pursuing her down the sidewalk long after having exited the open front door. 'They are definitely not my friends,' she finally admitted to herself, warm tears ruining her makeup.

Boycotting Surly Sam's Saloon and dumping her fake friends made for a vast improvement in Lynda's life. There was a marked upturn in her work at the research laboratory. Her creative and innovative abilities came to the fore.

Kevin had hurt her to the core by calling her a sot and a liar, plus he had encouraged everyone to laugh at her. Lynda could not just let it go. Somehow, she had to get even.

Lynda had never lied, but she had exaggerated a bit about the praying mantis being 15 feet tall, but how was she supposed to know different? People didn't walk up to one and tell it to hold still while they measured it. Isn't it enough to know that it is a **carnivorous** insect? The females are so mean that they eat the males after sex.

The more Lynda thought about Kevin, the more he irritated her. The thing to do was to prove to everybody that she was telling the truth. For that, she needed a 15 feet tall praying mantis. A daunting task for most people, however, Lynda was an experienced geneticist.

Gregor Mendel, the father of genetics, altered the size of organisms through selective breeding. That was nearly 200 years ago. Back then, it often took generations to get the desired results. Today, science has developed CRISPR which can produce similar results in a lot less time.

Lynda regularly used CRISPR in her work at the genetics lab, but it was usually in conjunction with a team project. No problem, Lynda was confident she could create a 15 feet praying mantis on her own in the privacy of her home. To start she would need to gather together some essentials, among which were the mantises gnome, a CRISPR kit, live insects suited to a praying mantis' diet, and a female *Phrygansis chinensis*, a more than two foot long walking stick insect recently discovered in mainland China.

Previous research had shown Lynda that the GH1 gene together with several variants determined the limits of growth. Nutrition was also important. DNA accounted for 80 percent of an organism's growth while nutrition was responsible for 20 percent.

Everything went as planned for the first three generations of Lynda's praying mantis experiment, but then she ran into problems. Ten foot tall praying mantises had to be housed in a chain link enclosure in her two acre backyard. As they grew taller, they thrived on a diet of insects and rodents. The food bill grew faster than the praying mantises. Also, their strong mandibles gnawed on the chain links, some of which appeared to be near the breaking point.

Lynda was having second thoughts about continuing the experiment. The mantises were beginning to resemble the creatures in the science fiction Sigourney Weaver movie, Aliens. She had a horrible nightmare about them and woke up the next morning determined to terminate the experiment, but when she went to feed the giant mantises, she discovered they had escaped into the National Forest that bordered her home. The north wall of the enclosure had been reduced to a mass of broken, twisted wire.

At twilight Ranger Dylan Peters was about ready to call it a day. And what a day it had been. Around 10 AM he had cited two men hunting deer out of season. After having been threatened by one of the hunters, he had removed the firing pins from both of their rifles. Dylan's three year old terrier, Pia, who put up a constant din of shrill non-stop barking during the incident, sensed something disagreeable about both men.

Then, as Dylan was about to break for lunch, his left back tire had a flat. Because the highway's shoulder was made of soft dirt, it had taken him an inordinate amount of time and energy to mount the spare tire.

Dylan was returning to the ranger station when he thought he saw someone or something enormously tall darting back and forth in a cluster of pine trees. By the time he made a u-turn and returned to the spot where he had seen the mysterious figure, it was nowhere to be found. Pia ran off barking into the forest, presumably she was following its scent. Dylan searched for her until dark but could not find her. Exhausted, he decided it would be best to wait for daylight before resuming the search. Dylan did not intend to discuss or write about what he had seen. Five years before a federal ranger had claimed to have seen Big Foot and even had a grainy photo of the

Sasquatch chasing a squirrel to prove it. After appearing on a few media late night talk shows, he was transferred to a lonely lookout tower halfway up Mt. McKinley, Alaska. Dylan did not want to join him.

Three days later, the residents around Lake Castaic awoke to find their small animals had vanished. In some cases gates were smashed, tethers were gnawed through, and sheds were flattened. Surprisingly, no one had heard it happen with the exception of 89 year old Tim Sullivan who claimed that space aliens corraled the animals together on the western edge of Lake Castaic prior to beaming them up to their spacecraft.

That night, a swarm of praying mantises, some as big as 13 feet, descended on Interstate 5, north of Castaic, blocking traffic in both directions. A terrier who was sitting on the driver of a recreational vehicle's lap, placed his front paws on the RV's dashboard and began to non-stop bark at a female praying mantis who was in the process of eating her mate. She paused to break the Winnebago's windshield and grab the dog whom she promptly swallowed. Soon, other praying mantises followed suit, smashing car windows and snatching small children from the backseats of vehicles.

The California Highway Patrol formed a wall of patrol cars in front of the northbound Interstate 5 lanes. Flares were shot in the air, illuminating a scene of carnage. CHP officers fired their shotguns into the swarm, killing many mantises, whose dead bodies littered the highway. But for every praying mantis killed, two more took its place.

The CHP lieutenant in charge called for reinforcements, but they were unable to get through. Mantises were unfolding their gossamer wings and flying to other points on the highway. There seemed to be no end to them. Then, at midnight, they disappeared as quickly as they came. It took four hours to dispose of the carcasses so traffic could get flowing again.

For eight days nothing was seen or heard from the praying mantises. It was thought that they were somewhere in the Los Padres National Forest. Then, on the ninth day, the swarm descended upon the Santa Barbara zoo where they ate the small animals and allowed the larger ones to escape. One person was killed and six were injured.

Lions, tigers, hippos, bears, snakes, buffalos, and rhinos roamed through the streets of Santa Barbara knocking over trash cans, scaring the bejeezus out of the community, and closing many businesses.

After watching CNN live coverage of the ongoing Santa Barbara disaster, California Governor Roberta Ruiz sent in the National Guard. In an unprecedented move, she also hired a fleet of DC-10 firefighting water tankers, filled them with a pesticide cocktail, and had them flown from their base in the high desert to Santa Barbara where plane after plane dropped its toxic payload on the swarm of praying mantises.

Mission accomplished. Men in bright yellow haz mat suits cordoned off the surrounding area and spent two weeks cremating mantis exoskeletons, neutralizing pesticide, and otherwise helping to restore the municipality's image. National Guardsmen rounded up the wild animals and returned them to the Santa Barbara Zoo.

CHAPTER 14

"Tastes like chicken," exclaims the freckle faced, sandy hair little boy in the television advertisements from Manna, Inc., the largest producer of genetically altered agricultural products in North America. "Have a second helping, it's good for you," advises his mother. The advertisement cuts to an animated cutesy chicken named Clara Cluck, who voices, "cluck, cluck, wholeheartedly endorsed by me!" This eighteen second commercial runs three times each primetime hour on all of the major networks.

Manna's synthetic chicken is made from the finest genetically modified grains and vegetables grown in the United States. You do not have to be a vegetarian to enjoy synthetic chicken, many people prefer it to the real thing. Not only that, but it is good for the environment. Plus it costs 60 cents a pound less. Isn't it what you should be feeding your family?

Evidently, lots of people thought so. In the first year it was introduced, synthetic chicken (aka faux chicken) captured forty percent of the market. Many fast food chains made the switch.

Then, in its third year of banner sales, a report by the Surgeon General linked synthetic chicken to stomach cancer. The Surgeon General's negative conclusions were quickly followed by articles in Lancet and other scientific journals identifying ingesting synthetic chicken as a major factor in developing intestinal polyps. Forty-two countries banned synthetic chicken imports. Manna's stock plummeted from a high of 679 on the DOW to its current low of 27. In an effort to bolster Manna's tarnished public image, Chief Executive Officer Chauncey Simmons agreed to do an interview with Robert Flash, host of PBS radio's "What You Need to Know" Morning Show.

Mr. Flash: "Our guest for this morning's show is Chauncey Simmons, CEO of Manna, Inc., whose plant based, genetically modified synthetic chicken has allegedly caused health problems ranging from intestinal polyps to stomach cancer. Mr. Simmons, how do you respond to that?"

Mr. Simmons: "Please understand that because the matter is being litigated there is a lot about which I cannot talk. I will say this, however, faux chicken is about as hazardous as gummi bears which, incidentally, is also produced by Manna, Inc. Their slings and arrows have no sting, I cannot help but sing:

Ich bin dein gummibar
Ich bin dein gummibar
Ich bin dein gummi gummi gummi gummi gummibar
Ich bin dein gummibar
Ich bin dein gummibar
Ich bin dein kleiner susser bunter dicker gummibar
Oh yeo
Ba ba bidubidubi jam jam
Ba ba bidubidubi jam jam
Ba ba bidubidubi jam jam
Drei mal darfst du beissen
Ba ba bidubidubi jam jam
Ba ba bidubidubi jam jam

Ba ba bidubidubi jam jam
Drei mal darfst du beissen
Bai ding ba doli party
Bamm bing ba doli party
Breding ba doli party party pop
Bai ding ba doli party
Bamm bing ba doli party
Breding ba doli party party pop
Ich bin dein gummibar
Ich bin dein gummibar
Ich bin dein gummi gummi gummi gummi gummibar
Ich bin dein gummibar
Ich bin dein gummibar
Ich bin dein kleiner susser bunter dicker gummibar
Oh yeo
Ba ba bidubidubi jam jam
Ba ba. . . ."

Mr. Flash: "Neither I nor most of our audience understands German. Would you please be so kind as to translate for our listeners?"

Mr. Simmons: "Basically, it all boils down to a message for Manna's persecutors."

Mr. Flash: "Which is?"

Mr. Simmons: "Bite me three times."

Mr. Flash: "Well, there you have it. Despite numerous scientific studies to the contrary, Manna continues to insist that synthetic GMO chicken is not hazardous to your health. There is a bill in Congress which would require labeling of all GMO products as such. As Chief Executive Officer of Manna, does that give you cause for concern?"

Mr. Simmons: "Not at all. We have been through this every Congressional Session for the past fifteen years.

Often, the bills either get pigeonholed or are killed in committee. Rarely, do any of them make it to the floor for a vote."

Mr. Flash: "All food producers are required by the Food and Drug Administration to list their product's ingredients on the packaging. Yet, on Manna's synthetic chicken packaging the only thing listed is 'Made in the U.S.A. from 100 percent organic matter.'"

Mr. Simmons: "The formula for faux chicken is a closely guarded secret. It's protected just like the recipe for Coca-Cola. Only two people at Manna, the CEO and the CFO, have access to that information. I can assure you, however, that we use only high quality, natural ingredients. At Manna, we care."

Mr. Flash: "You mean the finest genetically modified organic ingredients. That's a far cry from natural. Also, you did very little testing prior to marketing synthetic chicken and no long-term testing whatsoever. You are using consumers for guinea pigs. Have you no shame?"

Mr. Simmons: "I will not sit here idly and permit my character and the good name of Manna, Inc., not to mention the thousands of people who work for Manna, to be slandered by a ratings-seeking sensationalist. This interview has ended."

Mr. Flash: "Sensitive, isn't he? No doubt, the truth can offend. And here I thought that, being the host, I would be the one to end the interview. Anyway, we're about out of time, which I am sure Mr. Simmons knew better than me, since he is wearing a Rolex and the rest of us are fortunate if we can afford a Timex.

CHAPTER 16

When identical twins, Ricky and Randy Hewitt, graduated from High School in Mendocino, California, they began growing marijuana in state and national forests on a large scale basis. It was either that or flip burgers at MacDonald's. Considering the difference in the amount of money to be made, the choice wasn't hard to make. The main expenses were drip irrigation systems and camouflage netting. They reaped humongous profits selling cannabis to big city distributors. That is they did until cannabis became legal for recreational use. Licensing and taxing marijuana augmented the state's budget. Illegal blackmarket growers such as Ricky and Randy were being hunted down and prosecuted in an effort to protect California's revenue.

The Hewitt brothers' previous season's crop had been found and subsequently burned by state agents. Fortunately, for the brothers, the state agents were unable to trace the marijuana back to the Hewitts. Nonetheless, the agents had come too close for comfort. Ricky and Randy decided it was time to go legitimate and pay the state its exorbitant fees. However, that wasn't the end of it. Legal distributors and retailers paid top dollar for premium product from female plants with high levels of THC, which was what the carriage trade demanded. Low grade cannabis with stems and seeds, such as the Hewitts grew, often went begging. Buds were what the public wanted. For the right price, buds is what they got.

Clearly, the market had changed. Ricky and Randy searched through past issues of High Times magazine for something unique which would make their cannabis stand out from the competition. Ricky discovered an article on how to use CRISPR to increase the euphoria experienced by the marijuana smoker. It was all here, step by step, spelled out in detail, the recipe for a higher high. First, edit out two genes which are known to produce alkaloids from the peyote cactus plant and insert them into the cannabis gnome. Next, edit several genes known to produce hallucinogens from jimsonweed weed and attach them to the alkaloid chain. Add three protein producing genes from a morning glory seed. Voila!, enjoy the fruits of your labor.

The Hewitt brothers improved sinsemilla pretty much cornered the recreational marijuana market for the better part of a decade. Eventually, however, a number of other growers used CRISPR technology to develop stronger varieties. Genes from opium poppies and coca plants were edited into the cannabis gnome.

California cannabis overwhelmingly became the worldwide drug of choice. Independent growers merged into cartels. Drugs had become more of a social disorder than ever before. Complicit California was widely known as the narco state. It now has the fourth largest economy in the world. People having fake fun in the warm California sun.

CHAPTER 17

Doctor Maurice Moreau grew up idolizing Dr. M. Moreau, the man who was both his namesake and great-grandfather, the man whose ornately framed portrait hung directly above the tiled mantel in the spacious drawing room of the Edwardian mansion that he grew up in. One hundred thirty-five years ago great-grandfather had done ground breaking vivisection and surgery experimentation with animals and humans on his uncharted private island. The squeamish English called him a monster, while the French Academy celebrated his achievements. Upon his death at the age of 95, the French navy had purchased the island from his estate to use as a coaling station. The hybrid human animals he created were sterile. By the end of World War II they were no more.

Filling his great-grandfather's shoes would most likely be difficult. Following in his footsteps might prove even harder. He decided to take it one step at a time.

The first step was to attend and obtain a Doctorate degree from Aix-Marseille University like his great-grandfather before him, concentrating in paramedical sciences. That done, he needed to embed his name in the scientific community through significant, meaningful research and articles detailing his work published in medical journals. In fact, he did such a good job of it that medical scientists worldwide became familiar with his achievements.

Maurice Moreau was well into his fourth decade when he bought 150 acre Igoigori Island off the coast of Papua, New Guinea, telling his colleagues that from now on he would devote the rest of his life to research of his own choosing. "Why go to such a primitive, remote corner of the world with no mail service or internet access?" asked Professor Jean Bertran with whom Dr. Moreau had collaborated with on Cas9 CRISPR research. "Exactly, I value my independence. You know me well. In time it will all make sense," replied Dr. Moreau, embracing his good friend and colleague.

In preparing to move to his new home, Dr. Moreau gathered together the supplies he would need to survive since a supply boat stopped at Igoigori only when contacted by radio. In what may well have been an illegal transaction, he bought 150 live human embryos from California abortion clinics and 30 live embryos from spay and neuter clinics. Also, his laboratory equipment was crated and sent ahead of him.

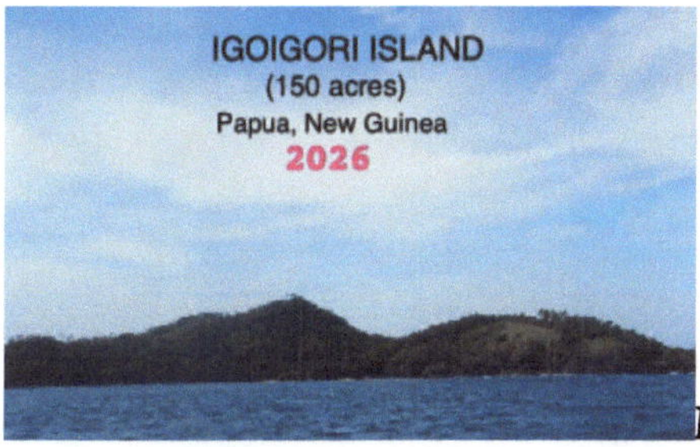

Maurice flew to Australia and then on to Papua. For the last leg of his journey he chartered a boat. Stepping ashore at Igoigori, Maurice was intrigued by the mangrove forest that choked the shoreline. Moving inland was difficult due to dense tropical foliage. He had forgotten to bring along a machete. Vines scratched exposed skin. It took him 45 minutes to walk 200 feet to the thatched enclosure that would serve as both his home and his laboratory for the immediate future.

It took a week to uncrate everything and set up his laboratory. Several glass flasks were shattered, along with some pipettes. It was hot and the humidity hovered near 100 percent. Mold and mildew might affect his research. Maurice made a list of things to order: bleach, petri dishes, and pipettes. An air conditioner would have to wait.

Great-grandfather Moreau kept detailed step by step journals of his experiments. His grandson read them in the evening by candlelight, fascinated by his great-grandfather's insight into animal nature.

Dr. Moreau was very much in need of an assistant, someone he could communicate with to perform the menial everyday tasks that were taking up far too much of his time. He could either recruit an assistant from Papua or create an assistant with CRISPR. He chose the latter.

Maurice began by severely editing a purebred Mastiff embryo, introducing genes that would form a human larynx, transform the paws into hands and feet, and provide an erect posture, in addition to substituting a human brain for a dog brain.

Dr. Moreau taught the resulting mastiff-human hybrid assistant to talk and perform chores. He named the creature Max. At nine months Max grew to 6 feet 3 inches and 180 pounds, but long before that Maurice bobbed Max's tail to make him appear more human. When waxed and shaved, Max could be easily mistaken for a human. Max slept at the foot of Dr. Moreau's four poster bed with the Moreau Family's Coat of Arms carved into the oak headboard. At night Max loved for Maurice to praise him while the master biologist rubbed his assistant's ears and chest.

Now that he had an assistant, Dr. Moreau was ready to delve full time into his research. He began by editing the gnomes of two creatures indigenous to New Guinea, a flaming red female eclectic parrot and a saltwater crocodile. Although parrots are capable of mimicking human speech, Dr. Moreau wanted to take the natural evolutionary process a step further, supercharging a parrot's bird brain with the addition of human brain genes. This resulted in a parrot who not only talked, but who really knew what he was talking about. In fact, the parrot learned to play chess and went on to severely critique the transformation of a saltwater crocodile from a sneaky, cunning predator into a highly intelligent super predator, claiming that such an action was unethical in that it could only result in increased death and destruction. Maurice did not particularly appreciate the unsolicited advice and constant interference in his affairs, so much so that he instructed Max to clip the parrot's wings, confining the loquacious bird to a perch in Dr. Moreau's laboratory.

When mature, the saltwater crocodile might measure 21 feet long and weigh more than 2,500 pounds, but for now he was able to fit comfortably in a 5 x 3 foot iron bar cage that occupied a corner of the laboratory near the parrot's perch. Max fed the juvenile crocodile raw wild boar meat and live jungle fowls. Igoigori Island had formerly been a sweet potato plantation, at least until the owner discovered that the island itself was worth many times more than all the crops that ever grew in its fertile soil. During the three years it took to find a buyer, wild boars took over Igoigori, uprooting everything in their path. Dr. Moreau taught Max how to set traps to catch the troublesome boars which when cooked on a spit over an open fire, gave them a break from the wild jungle fowl and fish they usually ate.

One day, while Dr. Moreau and Max were out hunting wild boar, the saltwater crocodile struck up a conversation with the parrot.

"Hey, Parrot, I saw you flying around the laboratory earlier today," observed the crocodile. "What gives? I thought Max clipped your wings."

"He did, but the flight feathers grew back," explained the parrot. "What's it to you, anyway?"

"I have an escape plan but I need your help to carry it out," pleaded the crocodile. "Please fly down here so we can discuss it. You can fit between the bars of my cage."

"No way!," screeched the parrot. "You intend to eat me. I watched as you stuffed yourself with live chickens. You are disgusting. This is one bird that isn't going to be someone's lunch."

"You have seen how much I eat. Why, someone like you wouldn't amount to an appetizer. What I value about you is your intelligence," reasoned the crocodile. "Without your help I would probably spend the rest of my life in a cage like some forlorn zoo crocodile. Sure, you could escape on your own, but how would you avoid being recaptured on this small, 150 acre, island? You need someone with my strength and intelligence to guard you until they give up and quit looking for you."

What the crocodile

"Turn around and take a look at the brass padlock on the door of this cage. You're bright, I bet you can figure out how to pick the lock," urged the sly crocodile.

The parrot had no sooner turned around to stare at the

lock before the toothy jaws of the saltwater crocodile closed around her. One swallow and she was forever gone.

"Burp-p-p," ripped the crocodile. Then he coughed up a mess of bright red feathers. "Curse that egghead bird," the crocodile said to no one in particular. "She gave me indigestion."

At twilight, Dr. Moreau and Max returned from hunting, bearing with them parts of a large boar. When they went into the laboratory to feed the saltwater crocodile the head of the boar that they had killed, they were shocked to find bright red feathers strewn about and no parrot to be found anywhere.

"Where is the parrot?," Max asked the crocodile.

"I don't know," replied the duplicitous crocodile, "one minute she was on her perch, the next she was flying around the laboratory, shedding feathers as she went. Maybe she flew the coop."

"You probably ate her," accused Max.

"The crocodile could not have ate her," Dr. Moreau intervened. "The lock on his cage hasn't been touched."

"I don't know how he did it," countered Max, "all I know is that the crocodile is the only creature on this island capable of committing such a vile act and then lying about it."

"You wound me deeply," said the crocodile with tears in his eyes. "I'm for the preservation of all intelligent life forms. That parrot was the one colorful spot in my dull, imprisoned life."

"I wasn't aware of your sensitive nature," commented Max. "When I fed you a chicken, you snapped at my arm."

"An unfortunate occurrence," explained the crocodile. "Being nocturnal, my day vision leaves much to be desired."

At breakfast the next morning Dr. Moreau and Max discussed the saltwater crocodile's future. "I don't trust the crocodile. It won't be long before he outgrows his cage," remarked Max. Dr. Moreau explained that his research on the crocodile was almost complete. After that Dr. Moreau planned to release the reptilian predator into the ocean. Igoigori wasn't large enough to support an adult crocodile. Most likely, the crocodile would then instinctively ride the ocean currents to one of the larger islands, much like a surfer rides a wave.

One afternoon, nearly two months later, Dr. Moreau told Max to bind the saltwater crocodile's jaws shut and tie a rope leash around its neck. Max led the four foot long predator to the spot in the mangroves where Dr. Moreau first stepped ashore. Taking precautions, Maurice shouldered a loaded 12 gauge shotgun to make sure that the predator wouldn't turn on them.

"Max is going to untie you and set you free; do not turn on us," commanded Dr. Moreau as he pointed his shotgun downward at the crocodile. As soon as Max cut the ropes that bound it, the reptile slithered down a bank into the tropical saltwater, tasting freedom for the first time in its life.

"I'm worried it will come back," remarked Max.

"No, it won't," declared Dr. Moreau. "I gave it the gift of life. To it, I am the Creator."

The saltwater crocodile floated with the current for two days without catching sight nor scent of land. On the third day, he spotted a native dugout. Coming closer, the crocodile saw an aborigine cast a fishing net into the ocean.

Paddling to the opposite side of the dugout, the crocodile stuck his snout out of the water and said in a loud and clear voice, "G'day mate. Here we are both at the mercy of the current and the waves, only you probably know where we are and I'm lost. Please point in the direction of the nearest landfall and tell me how far away we are from it."

The native fisherman looked all around, but could not tell where the voice was coming from. Then, seeing a portion of the crocodile's head surfacing at a distance, the somewhat nearsighted native assumed that a submarine had somehow become disoriented and was asking for directions. Standing up in the dugout, the aborigine pointed toward the south and shouted, "Ramu River, eleven kilometers due south!"

Not being a very good swimmer, the crocodile used his legs and tail to slowly paddle ashore. Approaching the Ramu estuary several hours later, the crocodile went ashore at a nearby cluster of mangroves and slept with one eye open until nightfall.

It was nearly midnight when the crocodile awoke. He was famished. Venturing inland on his stubby legs, he surprised a possum that was foraging on the ground and swallowed it whole. Hardly satisfying, an appetizer at best, he continued to hunt, but by daybreak he had only managed to locate two small rodents, one of which managed to get away.

Being a cold blooded reptile, he set out to sun himself on a rock at the edge of the Ramu River. It was a fatal mistake. Two crocodile hunters spotted him and low crawled through a grassy meadow to within 50 yards of the crocodile. A headshot dispatched the crocodile. The hunters had no way of telling that they had killed a partially human, intelligent crocodile, so they skinned and portioned it in the same manner they would have processed an ordinary crocodile.

The saltwater crocodile had always known he was destined to greatness. He was right. Part of his hide went to make a custom made pair of boots for a popular female singer and the rest to make a man-purse for a famous Civil Rights activist.

***

While the saltwater crocodile was drifting with the current at sea in search of a new island home, Dr. Maurice Moreau was busy concocting yet another experiment to demonstrate how geneticists could use CRISPR to improve the lives of the other animal species with which we share Planet Earth.

His was a noble goal, in step with that of his great-grandfather. Unfortunately, their well meaning experiments occasionally went awry, as was the case with the saltwater crocodile.

Dr. Moreau was deeply disturbed by what happened to the parrot. He knew that clipping a parrot's wings had to be performed periodically because feathers grow back, he simply had not realized that they would grow back so fast. Partly to assuage the guilt he felt in the parrot's demise, but mostly to reach a satisfactory conclusion on research that had been interrupted by an unexpected turn in events, Dr. Moreau went over the notes he had originally made on editing the parrot's DNA, made a few changes, and resumed his research as best he could.

One of the changes Dr. Moreau made was to use CRISPR to make the bird larger and heavier to the point where it could not possibly fly. Max reminded Maurice that a parrot needed to fly in order to get to the fruit that was a major part of its diet. "If we edit its genes to make it large enough, it will not have to fly in order to reach ripe fruit hanging in trees," responded Dr. Moreau.

Another modification was to substitute arms and hands with opposing thumbs for wings which would give the giant bird increased mobility and ensured the parrot could not fly. Dr. Moreau also decided to provide the parrot with sturdy legs. And the beak, which in a parrot is more suited to cracking open seeds than defending itself against predators, had to go.

If not a seed cracking beak, then what? Dr. Moreau thought long and hard about it. His assistant suggested a straight, general purpose beak, but Dr. Moreau nixed that idea. Ultimately, Dr. Moreau chose a raptorial/eagle beak so as to give the human/parrot hybrid a means of defending itself. Still, a number of scenarios of how the first parrot perished, each one worse than the last, crossed his mind.

Dr. Moreau, like many French men of his generation, was a misogynist. He thought of women as being the weaker sex. He could not permit what happened to the first parrot to occur again. This parrot was going to be a male. As if to reinforce his arcane views on gender roles, he chose to name his hybrid human/eagle parrot **Bruno** (meaning bear), which in Maurice's skewed view, was a name one would give to a ferocious pit bull or an East European thug.

It would not do to give Bruno an ordinary worm-like

parrot tongue. Although it took a while to get, Dr. Moreau thought it well worth the wait to acquire the forked tongue and poison genes from a spitting cobra. The combination of an eagle's flesh-tearing beak and a spitting cobra's forked tongue would definitely deter a predator. Adding poison glands capable of projecting nerve toxin four feet might even give Bruno the advantage in a fight to the death with a saltwater crocodile.

Do not confuse Bruno with Sesame Street's Big Bird. Despite the fact that they are both large, flightless, loquacious avians, the resemblance ends there. Big Bird is a muppet, nothing more than a man inside a bird costume. He is yellow, both in color and demeanor, whereas Bruno is an actual red feathered basher, a hybrid parrot capable of dealing with the meanest predator.

"I'm having trouble imagining how combining an eagle's beak with poisonous fangs will work," admitted Max. "Won't one get in the way of the other one?"

"Think of it as carrying a concealed weapon," explained Dr. Moreau as he bent over an electron microscope, supervising the editing of genes in the hybrid parrot's gnome. "If the beak fails to deter an opponent, only then will the parrot need to bring out the heavy weaponry. Remember, the hidden fangs are for defense. Bruno will be a non-aggressive omnivore with the ability to become a carnivore when sufficiently riled."

It takes long hours over many weeks of editing to create a hybrid parrot with the genetic makeup specified for Bruno by Dr. Moreau. Unfortunately, there can be errors. For instance, Max inadvertently spliced two crocodile genes onto one strand of a parrot DNA helix. Ordinarily, Dr. Moreau would catch any mistakes and correct them, but this time the error went unnoticed, a minor error which would later result in great difficulties.

Finally, the edited parrot DNA was injected into an edited human embryo which, four hours later, was inserted into an artificial placenta. The hard part was over, little to do now, but to wait, hope, and pray.

The embryo developed into a large egg inside a thick shell. Max removed the egg from the artificial placenta and placed it in an incubator. Thirty days later, the egg hatches. Due to frequent handling and close proximity, the hybrid parrot chick bonds with Max, regarding him as mother. Bruno recognizes that some parts of Max, e.g. the arms and legs, are similar to his own. Also, Max feeds the hybrid parrot chick by hand. The bond strengthens.

Twelve days later, Dr. Moreau gives Bruno a full spectrum of flash memory implants. Although not as effective as an actual education, they will suffice for the purposes of Dr. Moreau's experiment. Also, flash memory has the advantage of learning languages (in this case French and English) in an instant with a larger vocabulary than a student would have from twelve years of public school rote learning.

Bruno followed Max everyplace he went which resulted in some embarrassing situations, such as when Max relieved himself with Bruno standing nearby. It made Max extremely uncomfortable to be shadowed by what was within two weeks a one hundred pound hybrid human/parrot, always underfoot, constantly demanding to be fed. When Max brought up the subject one evening, Dr. Moreau explained to him how the bonding process works. Max determined to never allow himself to bond with one of Dr. Moreau's laboratory creations again. In the future he would be careful to distance himself as much as possible from newborns.

Bruno grew to be six feet tall and 200 pounds with scarlet plumage, resembling a National Football League linebacker wearing a red jersey. Most of the day, he followed Max around, coming much too close for Max's comfort.

One sunny afternoon, while Bruno was out foraging for fruit (the colossal parrot could strip a tree of its fruit in less than five minutes), Max mentioned to Dr. Moreau that he had seen Bruno tear apart a two foot long iguana with his beak.

"I was in the jungle when it happened," Max explained, "I don't think Bruno saw me. It was a grisly scene with blood and bits of flesh everywhere. Didn't you say he was a herbivore?"

"No, I told you Bruno was an omnivore with the potential to become a carnivore when riled," Dr. Moreau reiterated. "What you witnessed was most likely a subliminal response to an iguana's close resemblance to a saltwater crocodile. Such an instinctive response is to be expected."

"Something bothers me about Bruno," declared Max, "I cannot define exactly what it is, but it upsets me."

"I already told you, the poor fellow is convinced you are his mother, despite all of the evidence to the contrary. There is really nothing I can do about it other than to give you a sex change operation," Dr. Moreau chuckled while noticing a look of something between embarrassment and disgust flash across his assistant's face. Being rejected by one's mother can cause depression and do severe psychological damage. It can eventually result in suicide. Humor the lad, please, in the long run that way will cause less trouble. Trust me, I have lots of experience in matters of this kind."

In response, Max cleared his throat and turned away. He did not want Dr. Moreau to see how much he was hurting. Why was Dr. Moreau so concerned about Bruno's psychological well being, when he had so little interest in the psychological health of his assistant?

Dr. Moreau could see that he had taken the wrong tact with Max. He thought long and hard about what he could say to get their relationship back on the right track.

"I thought you knew you were running a risk of bonding with Bruno if you were too close to him when he hatched," remarked Dr. Moreau. "However, now I realize I may have skipped exposing your memory to the flash drive on bondingjn my rush to create an assistant to help with the workload. I fear I may have done you a grave injustice and I promise I will do everything I can to correct the situation."

The following morning, Max started wheezing and coughing. He was coming down with the flu. Dr. Moreau sent Max to bed and told him to drink plenty of liquids. He slept through the afternoon and only got up to go to the bathroom. Bruno was sitting in a chair next to the bed.

When Max went back to bed, he decided to clear up Bruno's misconceptions.

"I'm not your parent, I merely happened to be the closest one around when you hatched," Max revealed.

"I realize that. Dr. Moreau explained it all to me while you were sleeping," Bruno stated. "Dr. Moreau said you were my Creator, having made me from an edited hybrid human/parrot embryo. The bond between anyone and his Creator is unbreakable. It might be denied, but it is there nevertheless."

I really didn't have that much to do with it," Max remarked. "As his assistant, I was simply carrying out Dr. Moreau's instructions."

For the rest of the week, Max stayed in bed while he drifted in and out of consciousness, but every time he woke up there Bruno was assisting him in going to the toilet, eating meals, and taking medications. Max was gradually beginning to appreciate what Bruno could do for him.

"Dr. Moreau says we need to function as a family, relying on each other in our isolation on a small speck of land in the middle of a vast ocean," Bruno related to Max as he spoon fed him his breakfast of oatmeal and freshly squeezed Valencia orange juice. "If the world caught wind of what we are doing here, they might take it the wrong way. In fact, that is exactly what happened to Dr. Moreau's great-grandfather. The public was quick to rush to judgment. They called him a mad scientist and the hybrid human/animals he created as 'an offense against God.' No doubt these same otherwise well meaning people would call us 'abominations' and seek our immediate destruction. We can either stick together or hang alone. The chances of us being left alone to live our lives as we see fit are slim. I don't know about you, but I don't want to end up as the main attraction in a Freaks of Nature circus sideshow."

"Or worse yet, dead," Max responded. "I misjudged you. For that you have my apologies. We can't turn the clock back, but we can learn from our mistakes and try harder to get along."

Bruno nursed Max back to health in a week. Afterwards, they had a much improved siblings type relationship in which Max assumed the role of an older brother. In truth they shared genetic material, having been CRISPR edited for the most part to the same or similar specifications in the same way that humans and chimpanzees are 96 percent DNA related.

Bruno continued to prefer freshly killed raw meat to fruit. Iguanas supplied most of the protein in his diet. This was mainly the result of the two saltwater crocodile genes that had been accidentally spliced into his gnome. Eventually, Max learned to live with it in the same way that siblings learn to accept individual differences. However, Bruno's spitting cobra venom frightened Max until Bruno spit venom into the eyes of an enraged razorback boar that was charging Max. Thank God that Dr. Moreau had foreseen the need for Bruno's defense mechanisms. A jungle is no place for someone who is not equipped to defend himself. The weak and disabled are easy prey.

***

Igoigori was not as isolated as Dr. Moreau desired. Unwanted, uninvited visitors included various small fishing boats, small craft seeking shelter from a storm, and an Indonesian Navy patrol boat that circled the island three times prior to shelling it with six rounds from its deck gun (fortunately, nobody was hurt except for a few tree kangaroos on the northwestern coast).

Dr. Moreau normally dealt with intruders by ignoring them until they went away. His thatched domicile/ laboratory could not be seen from the shore and the dense jungle discouraged most from venturing inland. There was, however, one particularly notable exception when a party of Indonesian trappers in the lucrative business of supplying wild animals to zoos captured Bruno in a snare fashioned from a bent sapling triggered by tripping over a vine.

It was mid-morning with a heavy mist still covering Igoigori. Bruno was gathering medicinal herbs for Dr. Moreau when something suddenly snapped. Seconds later, he was hanging upside down, his head swinging back and forth inches above the ground.

As Bruno swung towards a trapper who was approaching him to cut him down and throw him in a cage, Bruno spat a stream of venom into the unsuspecting trapper's eyes. The trapper screamed in pain so loud and so long that Dr. Moreau and Max came running to see what was happening.

An advantage of being a parrot is that a parrot's head can twist and contort to reach any point on its body, giving it the ability to preen all of its feathers. Bruno twisted upwards to the point where he could cut through the vine that snared him with his eagle beak.

Bruno went berserk. He charged the other trappers, tearing apart their flesh. There were little bits of brains splattered on nearby trees. Blood was everywhere, forming puddles which the already rain saturated jungle floor could not absorb. By the time that Dr. Moreau and Max got there, the battle was already over. Bruno had cut the trappers into such small bits that it looked like they had been through a wood chipper.

"I didn't mean to kill them. I don't hate anyone," sobbed Bruno. "I was gathering herbs when suddenly something grabbed my right leg and flipped me upside down, hanging in the air. I pulled myself up and tore apart whatever was holding my leg. I fell to the ground and these strange fellows tried to stuff me in that cage over there. After that, everything was a bloody blur. I am going to prison, aren't I? Then, they will stand me against a wall, blindfold me, shoot me, and sell my limp, lifeless body to Kentucky Fried Chicken. I'll end up as Parrot McNuggets. Dr. Moreau, please save me!"

"Calm down," ordered Dr. Moreau, "dramatics won't solve our dilemma. Let's take our time and solve it one step at the time. Max, go back to the house and bring me a shovel and a rake. Bruno, go check the shoreline. See if you can find the boat that brought those intruders here. They would not be trapping zoo animals on a small remote island if they were licensed by the Indonesian government. I doubt if anyone will come looking for them. Nonetheless, we need to make it look as if they never set foot on Igoigori."

Several hours later, just as Max and Dr. Moreau were finishing cleaning up the site and burying the scant remains, Bruno returned, saying he had found a small sailboat on the rocky shore, covered with a tarp and some branches.

"Should I burn the boat?," asked Bruno.

"No, that will not be necessary," replied Dr. Moreau. "We can use a sailboat. Max and you can paint it a different color and alter its appearance as much as possible. With a sailboat we can pick up our own supplies and escape this island should it ever become necessary."

For the next six months, Dr. Moreau and his human/animal hybrid family lived in fear of people coming to search for the four dead trappers. Gradually, however, with the passage of time, the unfortunate incident seemed less important and life returned to normal. The weather beaten, clinker-built sailboat was painted bright red with the sails dyed red to match. Dr. Moreau wanted to build a small pier, but it would have to wait, as other matters took precedence. Two nearby smaller islets were to be explored, but first the refurbished sailboat had to be christened. A number of names were suggested, including *CRISPR Critters* and *Dreamboat Dregs*. In the end they settled on *Homo Aurelius* because the name foretold a bright future for humans and animals alike—a future which they were working to bring about.

None of them had ever crewed a sailboat before. Downloading articles from. the internet had of late become possible due to the advent of hundreds of small low orbit satellites bringing free broadband internet to anyone, anywhere on Earth. Dr. Moreau spent a week researching sailboating before they were ready to set out on their maiden voyage.

When they did finally set out on their initial journey, they spent their first few hours practicing setting a sail. Bruno got seasick. He spent the remainder of the day with his head hanging over the gunwale, ostensibly feeding the fishes.

They circumnavigated the first island they came to without finding a satisfactory landing. There seemed to be jagged rocks everywhere. Dr. Moreau decided it was not worthwhile to risk damaging the bottom of their boat. Besides, the island was less than five acres, mostly straight up and straight down.

They reached a second, larger island at sunset. The scene was breathtaking. The ocean, the island, the wispy clouds—everything was tinged in shades of red, especially their sailboat which shimmered in the half light. They pulled *Homo Aurelius* ashore onto a white sand beach that glittered in the moonlight. Since the night was warm with just a hint of a westerly breeze, they laid out blankets on the sand and slept on the beach. They woke up late the next morning and ate a breakfast consisting of iguana jerky and fresh papaya juice.

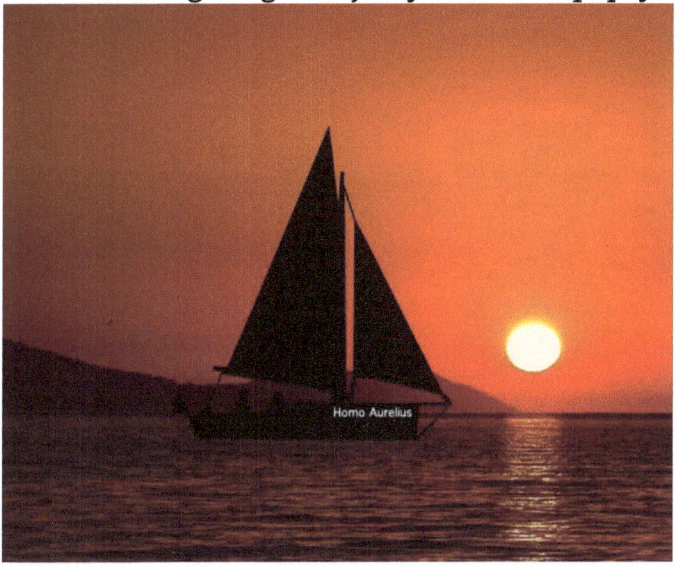

Delving into the jungle at the edge of the beach, they found bananas and mangos, two fruits which did not grow on Igoigori.

The wind had stiffened and was still blowing to the west. Dr. Moreau had Max and Bruno fill the sailboat with bananas and mangos, then refill their water bottles from a nearby stream. Dr. Moreau came across a "Private Property, No Trespassing" sign and decided it was time to leave. They launched *Homo Aurelius* at sunset and steered a course for home.

Sailing at night without any lights is the type of mistake that novice sailors might make, as indeed the first-timers that made up the crew of *Homo Aurelius* made, resulting in a large Japanese container ship cruising at 26 knots bearing down on the smaller vessel. In fact, if it had not been for an alert lookout on the bow of the *Kobayashi Maru*, the *Homo Aurelius* would have been reduced to kindling and its crew, asleep below deck, undoubtedly drowned. As it was, the wake of the container ship washed over the sailboat sending mangos and bananas over the side and nearly capsizing the *Homo Aurelius*.

The narrowly avoided collision happened when Bruno was supposed to be on watch. Max wanted to know why he had gone to bed without waking up the next watch.

"It was cold and wet and I was exhausted," Bruno confessed. "I tied down the rudder with a rope so we would stay on course before I went to bed. Neither man nor beast should have to suffer. We didn't come across any ships in the past two days. Then the container ship appeared out of nowhere and nearly ran us down."

"The waterways around Papua and the islands which surround New Guinea are relatively narrow," explained Max, "which is why we have to post a lookout at night. Last night, you were our lookout, but you left your post and nearly got us killed. Dr. Moreau is the Captain of this boat. When we are at sea, his word is law. All of us, including you, must obey his orders. I am the First Mate, the second in command. It is up to me to take care of the day to day activities aboard the boat. The big decisions are made by the Captain. Dr. Moreau is both our Creator and our Captain. Our survival depends on him. He is doing his best to improve conditions for humans and animals because we have to share Planet Earth. Similar to his great grandfather, Dr. Moreau's motives are largely misunderstood. The media prefers to portray him as a Mad Scientist, but we know him to be a kind, gentle, and caring soul.

Upon returning from their ocean excursion, Dr. Moreau suggested to Max that the sailboat needed a dock at which to tie up due to the frequent squalls and typhoons which struck Igoigori. It was to be small and well hidden from view. With Bruno's help it was completed in less than two weeks. In the interim, Dr. Moreau wrote two short articles, one of which suggested that endangered species might benefit from minor alterations in their gnomes which would make them better suited to changes in the environment. The other article served as a means of announcing that thanks to CRISPR new advances were in store for the entire Animal Kingdom.

Both articles were published in scientific journals four months later. It was the first time the scientific community had heard from him since he came to Igoigori. There had been rumors circulating that Dr. Moreau had gone to Moscow to conduct experiments on humans which would not have been permitted in any other country in the world.

Experimenting on humans had long been a flashpoint with the public and religious institutions. Often this included stem cell and embryonic research. And it definitely included cloning. It had become common to question the ethics, morals, and motives of scientists. Politics had come to the forefront and was now regulating what scientists could and could not do, similar to the way that the Inquisition hampered science during the Middle Ages. Is it any wonder that Dr. Moreau chose to endure the hardships and rigors of Igoigori rather than kowtow to Creationist principles?

Igoigori, however, was not as isolated as Dr. Moreau would have liked it to be. Every four months, like clockwork, an Indonesian Navy patrol boat (not always the same one) circled the island. Dr. Moreau had no idea about who or what the navy expected to find. Still, it bothered him, especially when a patrol boat's dinghy came ashore and shot two razorback boars before rowing back to the ship. Max reasoned that the patrol boat was most likely replenishing its meat supply. Dr. Moreau suspected it could be part of a regular surveillance of islands adjacent to islands claimed by Australia.

Typhoon Meranti struck Igoigori in 2016 with sustained winds up to 180 miles per hour. Fortunately, Dr. Moreau had advanced warning of the coming disaster. He had Max and Bruno take down the sail on the boat. They then dragged it 30 feet into the jungle, covered it as best they could, and secured it with rope to a cluster of trees. There was no saving the thatched roof on their domicile/laboratory. Still, the walls held. When the typhoon passed, they went outside to survey the damage. It was horrific. The jungle was flattened in many places and one-third of the dock had vanished. Dr. Moreau estimated that it might take several years for the vegetation to recover. CRISPR and the rest of the laboratory equipment were not damaged.

Dr. Moreau had Max post "Private Property—No Trespassing" signs at approximately 100 foot intervals along the periphery of the island. Although he had doubts about how much good they might accomplish, at least they could not do anything bad.

In the developing world the four illegal activities which generate the most money are 1. drugs, 2. Arms, 3. human trafficking, and 4. bush meat. It was the latter illegal poaching of endangered species which affected the residents of Igoigori the most. Bush meat was very much in demand in Indonesian markets. Boars, tapirs, bats, and monkeys were hunted periodically by the descendants of Indonesian pirates who had little to fear from law enforcement officers and environmental control officials.

It is estimated that more than sixty percent of the wildlife in Indonesia has disappeared in the last decade due to the ravages of fulfilling the demand for bush meat, supplying the fashion industry with exotic leather, and other banned activities. This even extends to butterflies, the rarest of which can fetch as much as $60,000 from foreign collectors.

Bruno sometimes woke up in the middle of the night and had a problem getting back to sleep. On those occasions he would go outside and eat fruit from trees until he felt sleepy. The last time he did so, he woke up at 2:30 A.M. on a hot night with no breeze. It felt good to go outside. Following a short search, he found a mango tree full of ripe fruit. Bruno was gorging on mangos and failed to notice an Indonesian hunting party who had come ashore to hunt bush meat. They had just killed a monkey when they came across what looked like a six foot, two hundred pound parrot with scarlet plumage. None of the hunters had seen anything like Bruno before.

"We can take that fat bird, the meat alone will go for a pretty penny," whispered the leader as the hunters snuck up on Bruno.

One of the hunters slipped a garrote around Bruno's neck. As the hunter was pulling it tight, Bruno sprayed his face with venom which burned his eyes and caused him to drop his garrote and scream. Rubbing his eyeballs only made the pain worse. Bruno's eagle beak slit the hunter's throat, putting the poor poacher permanently out of his misery.

The other hunters pulled back, except for the leader who shot Bruno between the eyes with an M-1 carbine. Bruno was dead before his body hit the jungle floor. The hunters then promptly butchered Bruno and packed the meat into two black plastic lawn bags. Then, they disappeared as quickly as they had come.

The next morning, Bruno was missed at breakfast. When he did not come to lunch, Dr. Moreau sent Max to search for him. It was not until two days later that Max stumbled across evidence that Bruno had been a victim of foul play.

"We should launch the sailboat and catch up with those evil hunters," Max suggested, "they murdered Bruno. They deserve to die."

"Yes, they deserve to die, and die they will, but I doubt that we will be the instrument of their death. Murderers have a way of killing each other off. Besides, we don't know what they look like and they have a three day lead on us," Dr. Moreau reasoned. "I am at fault. I confused remoteness with privacy. They really are two separate entities that often coincide but do not necessarily equate. I should have never bought Igoigori. We share few things in common with the Indonesians. It is us, not them, who should leave. Bruno will most likely be sold by the kilogram in the North Sulawesi bush meat market and I feel responsible. Tomorrow morning, I am going to put this accursed island up for sale, we are going to load CRISPR and the rest of the laboratory equipment aboard *Homo Aurelius* and search for a new home where there is a semblance of law and order and the local culture doesn't conflict with ours. I want to explore the islands on the Australian side of New Guinea until we find one that suits our needs. I cannot force you to come along, but I would like you, Max, to join me as a full partner in my grandfather's misunderstood mission to accelerate the evolutionary process, end the extinction of species, and share this planet equitably."

"I can't fathom most of what you are saying, but you are my Creator. You are a good man. I will follow you to the ends of the Earth. I have faith in you," testified Max. "I will always be at your side."

Bright and early the following day, Dr. Moreau put up Igoigori on an international real estate website as "For Sale." By noon they had loaded the sailboat with CRISPR and provisions. Max launched *Homo Aurelius* and set sail for the Australian half of New Guinea. Sailing with them were the hopes of an improved future for humanity and animals alike. We wish their enlightened endeavor success. The future of Planet Earth depends on it.

CHAPTER 17

In 2002, the International Criminal Court (ICC) was established in The Hague (Netherlands). The ICC has jurisdiction in crimes against humanity. Trials are conducted by a Tribunal. Criminals can be sentenced in absentia on the basis of documentary evidence alone.

Although the United States is not a member, the Centers for Disease Control, an American organization, was permitted to provide documentation and eyewitness testimony in the criminal case against Li Hong Fat (aka: "Mr. Spooky") whom it is alleged committed international mail fraud with malice aforethought in order to distribute a deadly virus throughout North America in which thousands were infected and hundreds needlessly died. Purportedly, Li Hong Fat, duped scores of underage females into acting as his agents.

Documentation was provided to the court by Dr. Owen Ostrowski, Senior Epidemiologist for the Centers for Disease Control, including several hundred affidavits signed by the minor girls and their parents or guardians.

In a unanimous decision, the Tribunal found Li Hong Fat guilty on all counts and sentenced him to 25 years in prison. A request was submitted to the Peoples' Democratic Republic of China for extradition. It is currently under consideration. In the interim, Li Hong Fat has been placed under house arrest in Wuhan, China.

Epilogue

I am not exaggerating when I say that CRISPR is making the largest biological changes in our species since *Homo Sapiens* first set foot on Earth. The same can be said for all plant and animal species. We have evolved to the point where we have assumed some of the creative functions that were previously the exclusive purvey of God.

CRISPR is a tool for gene editing. In the right hands it can create redder, riper tomatoes with a longer shelf life or put a halt to inherited diseases. In the wrong hands it can produce a pandemic. It desperately needs both pertinent legislation and effective enforcement. Do right and it will do right by you. I have faith that CRISPR will work to the benefit of mankind. It cannot help but alter the future of the planet. Science let the genii out of the bottle. Once out, it cannot be made to go back inside. It is only a matter of time until *Homo Sapiens* gives way to *Homo Aurelius* in the same way that Neanderthals gave way to Cro Magnons, but over a much shorter period of time.

Evolution is a hit or miss game of chance in which it often takes millions of years to see the results. CRISPR is a game of skill. Noticeable changes can be seen within our lifetime. Most likely, these changes will increase exponentially as time goes on.

Finis

Definitions

CRISPR - CRISPRs are specialized stretches of DNA. The protein Cas9 (or "CRISPR-associated") is an enzyme that acts like a pair of molecular scissors, capable of cutting strands of DNA. CRISPR can edit strands of DNA and RNA to add or remove genes much as a movie can be edited to add or remove scenes.

Antigenic shift - the process by which two or more different strains of a virus, or strains of two or more different viruses, combine to form a new subtype having a mixture of the surface antigens of the two or more original strains. The term is often applied specifically to influenza, as that is the best-known example.

eugenics - the science of improving a human population by controlled breeding to increase the occurrence of desirable heritable characteristics. Developed largely by Francis Galton as a method of improving the human race, it fell into disfavor only after the perversion of its doctrines by the Nazis.

genome - the complete set of genes or genetic material present in a cell or organism.

GMO - GMO, or genetically modified organism, is a plant, animal, microorganism or other organism whose genetic makeup has been modified in a laboratory using genetic engineering or transgenic technology.

variola major - There are two strains of smallpox virus. Variola major is the lethal strain, with a death rate of 30 percent.

variola minor - variola minor is the milder form of smallpox, with a death rate of less than one percent. Surviving infection from either strain provides cross-immunity, thereby having immunity to both variola major and minor.

Stem cells - are cells with the potential to develop into many different types of cells in the body. They serve as a repair system for the body. There are two main types of stem cells: embryonic stem cells and adult stem cells.

ocean gyre - a large system of circular ocean currents formed by global wind patterns and forces created by Earth's rotation. The movement of the world's major ocean gyres helps drive the "ocean conveyor belt." The ocean conveyor belt circulates ocean water around the entire planet.

Gregor Mendel (1822 - 1884), through his work on pea plants, discovered the fundamental laws of inheritance. He deduced that genes come in pairs and are inherited as distinct units, one from each parent. Mendel tracked the segregation of parental genes and their appearance in the offspring as dominant or recessive traits. Gregor Mendel was born in a German-speaking family in the Silesian part of the Austrian Empire (today's Czech Republic) and gained posthumous recognition as the founder of the modern science of genetics. Though farmers had known for millennia that crossbreeding of animals and plants could favor certain desirable traits, Mendel's pea plant experiments conducted between 1856 and 1863 established many of the rules of heredity, now referred to as the laws of Mendelian inheritance. Mendel worked with seven characteristics of pea plants: plant height, pod shape and color, seed shape and color, and flower position and color. Taking seed color as an example, Mendel showed that when a true-breeding yellow pea and a true-breeding green pea were cross-bred their offspring always produced yellow seeds. However, in the next generation, the green peas reappeared at a ratio of 1 green to 3 yellow.The profound significance of Mendel's work was not recognized until the turn of the 20th century (more than three decades later) with the rediscovery of his laws. Erich von Tschermak, Hugo de Vries, Carl Correns and William Jasper Spillman independently verified several of Mendel's experimental findings, ushering in the modern age of genetics.

Bibliography

Bergman, Mary Todd, "Harvard Researchers, Others Share Their Views," The Harvard Gazette, Jan. 9, 2019, Harvard

Fernandez, Clara,"Can Gene Therapy Become the Cure for Blindness," Labiotech.eu, Jan. 7, 2019, Berlin, Germany

Ledford,Heidi, "Quest to Use CRISPR Against Disease," Nature, Jan. 6, 2020, New York

Lofti, Melika, "CRISPR/Cas13 Therapeutic Option," PubMed.gov, Sep. 17, 2020, Washington D.C.

Pilger, Gerald, "The Benefits of GMO Corn," Country Guide, May 24, 2018, Canada

Straiton, Jennifer, "CRISPR vs. Covid-19," BioTechniques, Nov. 2, 2020, London, UK

www.ingramcontent.com/pod-product-compliance
Lightning Source LLC
Chambersburg PA
CBHW041132200526
45172CB00018B/8
9781636841816